To EmmA & Erick

Ether.   Three   science fiction stories

Andrew Roberts

Look Out For
my book On Madness
called 'Defeating The Voices'

GW00701529

Published by:
Chipmukapublishing ltd
PO Box 6872
Brentwood
Essex
CM13 1ZT
United Kingdom

www.chipmunkapublishing.com

High On Thoughts

As Thomas walked up the steps past the glass facade, steeling himself to enter the imposing facility, wind caressed his face and it carried the scent of the first flowers. It reminded him of a time when she was arranging flowers. There was no pretension as her body was naked, unashamedly so. She was unaware he was watching her. He imagined that her last breath lingered there, an empty pointless blessing. If Macey would never again feel a breath of wind, then why should he?

He remembered that from the first, there had been no hope for a cure, only a months-long lingering sense of dread, watching the beloved body shrivel and fade like last season's veined brown leaves crushed among the stones. She had died three months ago. Macey was truly, irrevocably gone.

Thomas Wrigley paused before the entrance, scared but determined to enter. He had caught a partial ghostly image of himself in the reflection of the entry door. He saw a tall, almost gaunt figure. The black wavy hair was stringy and nearly to his shoulders. His face was covered with patchy stubble, his over-large suit rumpled, and it seemed his socks did not match. Was he that inept? Well what did it really matter? He shrugged to himself, entered and took a seat in the waiting room and again wondered what it would feel like if he survived. He almost wished he could simply vanish, like she had. Maybe this was just an expensive way to commit suicide, if so, crying inside, he welcomed it. She had been such a giver of thoughts, high thoughts, crystal clear communication of love that he knew she would have rebuked him for his current display of weakness.

Within the lab, preparations proceeded. An assistant entered the aseptic room and said "Dr Whitson, are we certain we want to proceed with this Mr. Wrigley?"

"Why do you ask?" he appeared indifferent to the question.

"These psych-tests results... he is severely depressed. Is the group in such dire need of volunteers as to accept this level of risk?"

Dr Whitson sighed and wondered why he had to deal with such weaklings. Their risk aversion seemed to be a way of life these days. They had already had a successful three-week test run, forget about the previous failures. It was no secret that the group had lost some major funding, everyone was talking about it and the news was buzzing with it. "Technician, we will proceed. If you have a complaint you can go about it through the proper channels. The preparations continued and had indeed never stopped. The smell of ozone was strong in the lab. The sta-field generator enunciator floated in Whitson's view-plane, showing all systems were good to go. Everyone within view was working at a feverish but controlled pace with that nearly blank look that came from immersion within his or her own view panels. The staff were aware of the driving force behind Whitson's decision to place yet another guinea pig into stasis. No one talked of the crisp failure, in a shallow grave, apparently successfully concealed from the media.

"Thomas Wrigley, please proceed to waiting room seventeen." The listless voice of the pale nurse intoned. Why did he suddenly feel chilled? There seemed to be no strength in his legs as he wobbled slightly, like a sail suddenly bereft of wind.

"Is something wrong? Do you need help?" she asked, showing a little more life, apparently waiting to pounce on a moment of weakness.

Eyes widening in spite of a desire to hold back any emotion, but fooling no one, he said "No. I'm fine. Must have been a slick spot on the floor." If he did not get to a bathroom first, there might really be something in the floor, he had not realized until this moment how full his bladder was. Worse, he knew that in the inner room his family would be waiting to say what could be a final good-bye.

Though the temperature inside the lab was too cool, Thomas had to keep wiping the moisture from his face and neck. He tried to pry his eyes off his loved ones, wondering in his heart if he would see them again. Would they miss him like he ached for Macey? If he survived, how would he feel about them if they all died in the intervening years?

"Thomas, are you sure?" Dad's usually deep voice quavered with sorrow.

"Yes, I'm sure - now stop asking." It was difficult enough.

"Don't you know that we will almost certainly be gone by the time the years are up?"

Of course he knew. "We've been through all this! It is my choice, I know the risk! No-one can stop me."

The farewells were over, and he allowed rather than assisted the medical ministrations and subtle indignities upon his body by the nurses, doctors, and technicians. Squeezing back the tears, he knew the hugs and kisses from his parents and brother would haunt him. Suddenly the resolve to travel fifty years into the future seemed galling, unnatural and horrible. But his deep sadness, mingled with a spark of desire to see that future, to learn about it, to live as one of them - was a project and a journey that he felt compelled to take.

With his personal view-plane deactivated, the network was gone. As darkness enveloped his senses, his last thought was a wonder if his meager investments would even keep pace with the times as a provision to sustain his young-old self if or when he awoke.

On waking he discovered a team of scientists looking over him who were in turn being watched by a team of elderly people. "Welcome to the year 2052 young man, how do you feel?" His first thought was a bit hazy but it was something like 'thank God, I made it'. He tried to move and found his body unwilling or unable to move. They had stimulated his muscles over the fifty year period but there was still some atrophy.

It had taken Thomas a full week of intensive physiotherapy before he could fully walk again which he found hard to deal with along with the press coverage he had received. After two weeks of being prodded and tested he was finally released into the new unknown world.

When he walked out of the building he found a handful of reporters and a white haired man who he could just about recognize as his brother David. "Congratulations brother you've finally arrived. I always told you this was a strange idea."

They went back to David's house inside an air car. "This is about the biggest surprise you'll encounter in the world today. Only the rich can afford these toys. It's not just an ordinary petrol engine but a hybrid, using solar power when the sun's out and electricity and petrol at other times. The cars can travel through the air on satellite roads which means you can't crash into someone coming the other way because you are on a prearranged flight path. It does however give you enough leeway to overtake. Also the faster you wish to go the higher the flight path so that when you near your destination you go lower so as to find the place and not hold up faster traffic."

Thomas looked around his brother's house and noticed his bonsai trees.
"Wow, the trees are amazing Dave, you've done really well with them."
"Yes a couple of them died but the rest thrived pretty well."
"Thank you so much."

After settling in to his new surroundings within a week he was looking for a job. He eventually found one as a waiter in a restaurant and quickly picked up the way of handling the electronic waiters pad that were in standard use.

Eventually he became friendly with a lad called Sid Withers the Head Chef and was glad of his company on the days off since his brother was a great deal older than he was and Thomas wished for company more his age.

On one of the days off Thomas had been introduced to a new gadget that had not long been developed. "This is a brain wave amplifier and

receiver" announced Sid with what seemed to be a great deal of satisfaction. "The wearers of this device are able to telepathically communicate basic emotions." Thomas had heard of this device from his brother. It was mainly used by the younger generation, mostly to make sex more of a two way thing. Sid explained," this thing has got great potential Thomas" and then he whispered excitedly "have you ever done any acid".
Thomas said "no but I've always wanted to try it." "Well these two coupled together are the best thing since sliced bread, if you haven't tried them you haven't lived." Thomas replied "Well what are we waiting for?" As if rising to the challenge.

They took the acid tabs and waited for the onset. After half an hour or so they began to put the headsets on whilst giggling uncontrollably. They were in hysterics before long and enjoying every minute of it. Gradually Thomas's mind began to flit from one thing to the next and soon became very scatty. Thomas couldn't believe the strangeness of the drug. Everything seems to be very intense, including emotions. Colours seemed to be very bright to the eye. He could sense Sid's own brain undulating in an endless stream of emotions and at this Sid began to laugh again as he realized that Thomas was curious as to what Sid was feeling. Then their retinas locked and Thomas slid down into the tunnel of Sid's eyes and they both began to laugh. He could feel him walking around in his skull. The laughing grew louder and seemed to echo in Thomas's mind until he started to think he was laughing at him. At this Sid stopped laughing and for the rest of the trip Thomas tried his best to enjoy it. However, deep down he didn't enjoy being out of control with respect to his mind and seemed to develop a form of mental claustrophobia. He could feel the drug gradually close in on his mind.

Eventually Sid said goodbye to Thomas and warned him to take it easy because he was especially mentally vulnerable on the comedown. Sid had thought it was perhaps a bad idea to have said goodbye to Thomas and that maybe it would have been better to have sat with him a while but Sid thought about this a while and eventually shrugged, said to himself "don't worry about it" and went to make a cup of Tea. Sid was that sort of person. The sort that could just neck trips like candy and not let anything bother him.

Thomas on the other hand was not like Sid. He could not straighten out his mind and was starting to feel emotionally exhausted. He could see a man walking towards him from up the street he wasn't sure but it looked like a policeman. At this point he began to get nervous, he wasn't sure why but he started to think that he was walking in an over relaxed way so he tried to walk like he was going somewhere. At this point he noticed that it wasn't a policeman but a business man, but even then he found himself being paranoid the closer the person got to him. "He knows I'm tripping" he thought to himself. Pretty soon he became paranoid about any people that came near him.

After a brief interlude of feeling like a zombie Thomas realized he was still not free of the drug and decided to walk. "walk anywhere to get some air" he thought to himself. As he walked he found he was lost but he didn't care. Town had changed a lot in fifty years and this thought seemed to relieve him of the mental constraints momentarily. He heard bells from around the corner and as he approached he could tell it was coming from a United Reform Church, except he could tell they were not the usual bell sound. They seemed more crisp and almost electronic,' that was it' they were electronic and he pondered on this for a while realising that it must be a sort of statement by the church that they were willing to move with the times. He crossed over the road and noticed some new shops. Well not new but to him they were new. He noticed the Cyber café where the students hung around drinking coffee and smoking cannabis.

The acid was doing some strange things to him. It was like being on a sea of acid, paddling for dear life with no sight of dry land. It was all consuming and introspective.

Thomas was beginning to recover and wished for sleep and so after recognizing where he was he headed for his brothers home.

Thomas was the sort of person that thought about life deeply. He would spend a lot of time thinking about where the human race was headed and he worried about the future of mankind. He realised that the next century or so was crucial to the continued existence of man. The reason for this was that technology and industry were raising the stakes with regard to pollution and its effect on Mother Nature. There were deadly diseases like aids and biotechnology companies were producing new species of plants and animals that were resistant to bacteria and insects and were changing the food chain greatly and worst of all, these changes were to some extent permanent. He used to worry about the effect of modified DNA in the food chain and whether or not it affected our own DNA. After all they say that you are what you eat. At the same time as raising the risk of damaging our way of life forever, there were increased benefits. For example, in order to guarantee the continued existence of man then he would have to reach for the stars. In other words once another planet was colonised there would be much less of a risk of total annihilation. While we were still on Earth we were in real danger from biological, nuclear and chemical weapons or even CJD, the human form of mad cow's disease in the 1990's, of which the amount of cases was now in the thousands. Thomas would feel apprehensive about all of these things and would sometimes get depressed, believing that mankind would not make it through this difficult time.

He started to worry more and more about what was happening in the world and felt he was the only one that cared.

As the weeks passed Thomas began to notice something peculiar. People seemed to be behaving in odd ways and to start with he could not put his finger on what it was. Human speech seemed to contain almost subliminal meaning behind a facade of words. Even his brother seemed to be unusual and cagey, as if he was trying to hide something. As if he had stumbled across something he shouldn't have. Eventually it occurred to him what the answer was and as soon as he saw   became as plain as the nose on his face and he could explain this new form of behavior because of it.

That day he had a visit from his old friend Johnny. He was seventy two now and showed every bit his age. Johnny sat down and said "so how you do like this point in time is it so different from before."
"Johnny why didn't you tell me."
"Tell you what."
"that people are becoming telepathic."
"oh you mean the brain wave amplifier and receiver. That's just a play thing it doesn't have any practical applications."
"No I don't mean that" said Thomas earnestly "I mean people are becoming telepathic for real."
"What are you talking about Tom? Are you off you're rocker?"

It was apparent that Johnny was not aware of this new phenomenon. What followed was a heated argument on the matter, for Thomas was so adamant that this telepathy existed.

Thomas tried to gauge how many people knew about this effect. He found it to be in most modern music although for some particular reason nobody came out and directly said it. He discovered that some politicians were capable of it judging from their mannerisms on the Television. He even tried to communicate with some of them on live TV, with limited success.

He noticed that the waitress at his place of work was virtually controlling the restaurant workers. Even the restaurant manageress was doing the leg work while the waitress just stood there content with polishing spoons and coercing others to do different jobs.

He sat in the bar area on his lunch break and tried to raise and lower the noise level in the pub with some success.

Thomas noticed that generally younger people were better at telepathy than older and more of them were aware of it. He figured that this was because a young mind is more supple and open. Wherever he went he found that some people knew and some didn't. Thomas noticed once an old man in the park sweeping the pavement and his face was twitching with stress. Thomas realised the man was perhaps a little disturbed about how the world was these days. The man had obviously realized that something was different about the world but didn't quite know what and Thomas feared that he would never click on because his mind was closed and it would never open. He thought it was sad that he would never know about this new form of communication. Thomas could tell all this just from his facial expressions and reading his thoughts.

Thomas was beginning to see who knew and who didn't. Telepathy was occurring in patches and pockets, the people who did know were urgently getting on with their lives and the people who didn't know were going through major stress caused by a combination of the effects telepathy and ignorance.

Some businesses were embracing the phenomena by only employing young people who knew and others were shunning it using mainly old people. Others were blissfully unaware of it and still others had desertion in the ranks where youngsters were wiping the floor with their bosses. Some businesses sent out subliminal messages to entice customers into their establishments. The people who didn't know seemed like sheep being led to do whatever the people in the know wanted.

As time went on he become more and more obsessed with the idea that people were becoming telepathic. He tried to alter the trade levels of the restaurant and found that one night when he was filling in as a starter chef and he tried to increase trade that night. Within an hour he was inundated with orders and was incapable of working at the given pace. Consequently the assistant manager had to come in and bail him out.

Members of the government were beginning to notice this telepathy and looking back he found that the first person to notice this was Margaret Thatcher, a Prime Minister from his own time. It seemed to give a reason for her hard nosed approach to the problem of telepathy and the general urgency of governmental matters. This was the reason for the next government's philosophy of 'back to basics' with John Major. In other words people and businesses were getting hysterical and this slogan was designed to prevent that panic. Things soon began to take on a feeling that judgment day was on its way.

He found that he couldn't seem to master the art of telepathy and as time grew on he became more introverted, too cynical to speak and more weary from the frustration.

Johnny had often called him on the telescreen and eventually they fell out, with Johnny saying "why do you insist on this obsession? Why do you keep saying things that aren't true?"
"I can only tell you how I see things, Johnny, and that is how it seems."

"Well I'm sorry Thomas but I've had a belly full, goodbye."

Thomas found more and more increasingly that he couldn't control this. He found that his brain was beginning to leak thoughts and it was becoming an involuntary thing that was taking him over.

He realized that children were better at telepathy than adults and because the parents could not see this telepathy happening and the kids didn't understand this it started to send them into their own little world. This in turn was causing many adults to take their children to doctor's psychiatrists and psychologists. Even Thomas's boss at the restaurant was having problems with his unruly son.

Thomas had only ever met one man who seemed to be doing well in the world and was using the effects of telepathy to his advantage. This was one of the assistant managers, Nick, at the restaurant. He was a very funny chap who was well liked. However, there seemed to be an anterior motive about this young man that he couldn't quite put his finger on. "He must be using some aspect of telepathy that he hadn't thought of" Thomas thought to himself. One day Nick was talking to Thomas,
"While you're here Thomas keep you're head down and work hard. Work hard and play hard, and while you're at it stay off the drugs. That Sid is a bad influence on you."

Eventually Thomas began hearing voices inside his head. At first one or two words and then gradually the voices, coming mostly at night while lying in bed, grew louder and more and more voices joining in until eventually he could hear thousands of voices in an endless babble that was almost unbearable.

People were picking up on those leaking thoughts unconsciously and despite trying to progress further with the company he found he was not doing very well.

His brother David had many talks with him about this obsession. He was very analytical about it and eventually he said "I think you should get help Thomas."
"Why?"
"Because you need help"
"Rubbish, it's just something I need to understand, That's the way it seems to me."

But as time went on and Thomas found his head leaking more and more and the voices growing louder then the more he considered David's offer of help. He realised why people were not saying anything about the telepathy because it became unbearable once known about and ignorance seemed like bliss. He eventually found that alcohol seemed to lessen the backward effects of the telepathy and seemed to relax the brain a bit so it didn't leak so much and the voices became silent and Thomas soon became a heavy drinker, sitting in the pubs with all the other people who "knew". Of course, Thomas thought that Assistant Manager was a heavy drinker and he often played drinking games at night with most of the staff. That must have been his secret of success. Ply the staff with alcohol and thus prevent the ones that don't know from realizing and reduce the amount of stress (caused by the telepathy) in the staff who do know, creating an efficient workforce.

It soon became apparent that the pub trade would very quickly become one of the most important trades due to this fact and Thomas had repeatedly tried to further himself in this trade before the real confusion throughout the world set in. In fact Nick had studied Economics at college and got a first degree honours. He must have known that about this trade being a hot tip. Come to think of it Nick had been promoted something like 3 or 4 times since he'd worked for the company. Thomas on the other hand was not progressing at all well and started reading the jobs section of the paper each week.

Thomas gained an interview with a Hotel and Restaurant in another town nearby. The interview wasn't too bad but it was like a game of cat and mouse. He didn't know if the manager knew or not. Sometimes he would see deep wisdom in his eyes, as if he'd known for years, and at other times he seemed completely innocent of what was going on. The man was Egyptian so Thomas began to consider what other countries might know of it. He figured that Egypt was not as advanced technologically but they were definitely more advanced spiritually. Had his people known for decades or even centuries? Thomas decided not to try and read his thoughts or coerce him at all as this was probably not what the manager was looking for. At the end of the interview the manager gave him a knowing smile that caught Thomas off guard and took this to mean that the manager did know.

Eventually he gave in to his brothers' plea and was referred to a Psychologist. On the day of the appointment he had arrived early and was soon ushered in to the Doctors room where a large calm man said please take a seat Thomas and tell me what has happened to you."
He tried to tell the Doctor through fits of tears and when it was over he felt as though a huge weight had been lifted from his shoulders. Having said this he still felt that a bit wary of his Psychologist because he was unsure as to who he could trust and whether or not this would go down on his records. He did not know who had access to these records.

"There is no doubt Thomas that you are experiencing what is known as a Psychotic Episode. This was bought on by the acid you had taken with you're friend. A great many people who get Psychosis tend to think they are Psychic but don't worry; with the right drugs we can treat it."

Thomas had sat in the smoking area of the hospital after the injection and considered what the Psychologist had said. Maybe this Psychotic Episode was just a form of Psychic Overload when people become operant telepaths maybe this fate is what happens to all telepaths, Thomas felt let down by society for allowing such a wonderful ability to become lost and shunned by all around and for no one to actually check out his claims. After all telepathy could occur, most people think that some sort of physical exchange has to take place, like brain waves, but it doesn't if you can accurately predict what someone's thoughts can be because by following logic a form of communication can occur once your mind has allowed that communication to happen. People can already predict some peoples thoughts to some degree and when some sort of threshold of understanding is reached then telepathy will be allowed to occur. After all there are patterns to chaos just as each individual snowflake has its own pattern. It would be like a more advanced form of empathy. Also, the laws of physics seem to echo this. Schrödinger's cat states that just by observing something it can affect the nature of objects. If Schrödinger's box is not opened then the cat is neither alive nor dead, until it is observed. This illustrates that our minds interact with the environment. Thomas rocked slowly backward and forward as he pondered on this a while but as he felt the effects of the injection come on his thoughts became lost.

Two years after Thomas's psychosis he wrote a book based on his experiences and perceptions and because so little was known about psychotic experiences yet there was a lot of interest in it, he made quite a lot of money from it. Through writing about his experiences he found that he could distinguish between obsession and reality but it had before just felt like a good and bad dream all rolled into one whereby sometimes he would prefer the psychic world and other times the normal world. If Thomas ever felt those two worlds start to converge again then that would mean a relapse and that was the last thing Thomas wanted. He found writing therapeutic.

Since going through this psychotic experience he found it had changed him. He realised that worrying about the future of mankind would not do him any good as you can't do much about it. He found also that he was less pessimistic about the future and was in fact feeling quite positive about the future. It was as if he had to go through this ordeal to come out the other side a better person. "there but for the grace of God go I."

With the money he had earned from the book he decided to go back to the suspended animation organisation and travel forward again for another Twenty years. He felt he still needed to know more about the future and where Science and Technology were headed and science fiction failed to provide this, he felt that he just had to keep going further.

He had paid the suspended animation organisation to provide him with the necessary accommodation after the suspension and for twelve months there after.

So once again he was put into Suspended Animation and by this time the firm had just about perfected this form of time-travel so there was little or no ageing.

When he came out of storage and was now living in the year 2101 he found that a great surprise awaited him.

The brainwave amp and receiver which had been developed in the 2040's had been given a major boost five years ago. These telepathic implants, as they were called, were designed to learn how each individual brain worked and as the wearer continued to learn how best to use the device the same also occurred with the implant, learning how best to interpret commands from the brain, a sort of ultimate personal computer that could instantly talk to any other personal computer at any time. You could also mix your dreams and nightmares with other people. The receiver could access the internet at any time as well and people had their own curriculum vitaes displayed at their own individual websites, but not just one CV but several of them so they could choose which one to submit to different people. For instance, a different CV would be used when going to parties from meeting people at work. Some people took this new CV writing very seriously and it soon became an art form and others took it as an opportunity to be whoever they wanted to be and wrote nothing more than a string of lies or alternatively if they so desired they could just write a poem about squirrels. That was the advantage of the system you could use it to create whatever first impressions you liked with the benefit of being able to plan what information you allow a person to know. With this in mind, a person could find out about anything at anytime of the day or night so long as it was on the internet, which did in fact cover just about any subject possible because by this time the internet contained almost three times the amount of information as the sum total of all previous knowledge. With being able to access this information any time it meant that previously wasted time, spent say in the shower, toilet or driving were put to greater use and people were thus given the opportunity to learn more about the world and, subsequently, life was speeded up greatly. Nearly every person had their own personal web site with every aspect of their lives and this could be accessed by others so that at times when you first meet someone and want to know more about them then you could do so unobtrusively and decide whether you wished to speak to them.

The Implants could be designed to perform several different tasks. Firstly the device could communicate with other implants over short distances of about 30 meters. Secondly it could 'roam' over longer distances of up to 300 Km, although research was proving highly successful in lengthening this distance. The roaming mode worked a bit like a mobile phone connected straight into your neurons. Thirdly, the device could be programmed to transmit only conscious thoughts at will.

Thomas used yet more of the money from his book to have an implant programmed to telepathy.

Of the current population about fifty percent had the implants. These groups were mainly the youngsters who had quickly recognized the advantages of a population that had access to people's minds where there would be no misunderstandings about anything. However the older generations were a bit more skeptical about having ones thoughts broadcast to any old person.

Some businesses took up the technology and others didn't. Firms such as supermarkets and restaurants or anywhere that needed to keep in close contact with their staff only took on people with the implants. Some people were faster at communicating than others so the scenario that Thomas falsely perceived in the restaurant where the waitress was controlling the manageress was not so far from the truth after all. Thomas felt like he'd been given a preview of the future with his psychotic experience and he felt glad to have experienced it. He asked himself if his fantasy world and reality were colliding again and worried about going mad again.

Because of this new form of communication the younger generation learnt to use telepathy to their full potential and eventually began to communicate in a faster way by transmitting images rather than words. This was a much faster form of communication and served to greatly increase the pace of life much the same as cars managed to increase the pace of the previous century.

However the new imagery form of communication served to put a division between the young and the old. The older generation became frustrated with the youngsters who would often end up finishing sentences for them. At the same time the youngsters were proud of their trendy way of communicating because it had street credibility. The elders labeled them uncouth brats who had lost any form of subtlety to this new invention. Therefore this form of communication, which was a met cognitive tool, or a brain amplifier, which allowed information to pass into the head faster than anything that had gone before consequently allowed for a faster form of thought that led to a more sophistication of the mind. Other forms of frustration quickly arose from the device which

Thomas thought was the best thing to come out of this unfamiliar century.

Technology had also advanced in other areas such as genetic engineering and people could now get babies that were free of hereditary diseases on the National Health Service or alternatively they could get genetically enhanced babies that were superior in both looks and intelligence from other humans. However, some people still preferred the traditional method of making babies so that their genes could be propagated. Other areas of the human DNA were being experimented upon and it was believed that the senescence gene, which aged people, could be isolated and would not be within the DNA of future generations (it was believed that the top limit for our bodies would be 140 years), however this research was far from being perfected and because it was so complicated would not be around for some years.

One time Thomas was shopping and he noticed a man complaining about an item of clothing he had bought, to a sales girl. He was talking very politely to the woman about what the problem was and at the same time he was screaming telepathically various obscenities at the girl who was becoming quite flustered.

Similarly while driving Thomas began to notice that few people were polite when on the roads and the majority of people were shouting insults to each other for even the slightest provocation. Thomas began to notice that this was prevalent everywhere with people being very basic and scathing in their telepathy.

After some months of living in this new society Thomas noticed that more and more people were dropping out so to speak. Many became depressives due to all the negative stimuli being received, and still others dropped out of society through choice and often turned to drugs. There was a great backlash towards technology and a music revolution that put the 1960's to shame. Thomas didn't much like this time which he had previously thought was a God send. Consequently he decided to use what little money he had left from the book he had written to go back to the suspension firm, which still existed and was now thriving off of hippies and a popular religious cult and also many ordinary people who were disillusioned with the times. The religious cult known as the Gestalt, meaning the whole is different from the sum of its parts, philosophers believed that when the whole world became unified under telepathy then the second coming of Christ would arise and he or she would set forth a new consciousness that would mean listening to the voice of nature, Gaia.

He decided to go forward another nine years as this was all his budget would allow because of the inflated prices due to the suspension organizations popularity, although the conglomerate did in fact give him a special deal because he was one of the first to test out the service.

After the Physiological examination and exercises was over he realised that he had no place to stay and as he had no living relatives to stay with he would have to live rough for a while. He had spent the night on a park bench and as he stirred he felt a faint breeze on his face and lifted his head to get some of the fresh air from this new year of 2111. A man was walking his dog on the pavement as he looked up and Thomas asked the man what the exact date was and the time. The man looked at him quizzically, not able to comprehend, then followed a rather long telepathic inquiry in which, Thomas realized, the man had so politely slowed down his thoughts and used words instead of images. The man finally understood Thomas's situation and informed him that the date was now the 10th of December 2111 and the time was 7.35 am. As Thomas sat up, the man, almost instinctively, took a seat next to him and began to talk to Thomas in speech as he felt it might be a bit rude to head talk a guy originally from the year who was born in the year 1971. Thomas noticed that the mans dog was broadcasting images of food to both him and the owner with a forlorn look in his eyes. Thomas was delighted with the idea that animals should be given the capacity to talk in this new way.

While walking through town he noticed how mentally polite people had become. It seemed that after several years of people mentally shouting at others they had finally calmed down and learnt to use the device without sending people mad.

As Thomas was walking through the main street of the town he noticed a juggler busking for money. She was juggling with five balls in the usual way but Thomas noticed there was a major difference. She was actually demonstrating the speed at which a person could communicate using thought patterns and the balls had a direct relationship with the juggler's thoughts which was plainly visible to onlookers. The artist would make cheeky comments to people in the crowd and she would occasionally be heckled by individuals in the same way that a traditional entertainer would be. The only difference was that the communication was much faster and more complex. So much so that Thomas was hard pressed to keep up with the flow of communication. It was plainly obvious that people who had grown up with this new form of 'mobile phone' were much quicker at talking.

Thomas pondered on this fact for a while. It seemed like an inevitable effect of technology. Just like blackboards had speeded up thoughts and the ability to communicate so had computers, and now the implants had speeded communications up. Just like a mathematician who had spent all his life working out equations on the blackboard could therefore both communicate and think a lot faster in his chosen field. His consciousness had learned to expand and get faster in this area. Similarly, the juggler had learned to think in terms of images with more and more detail in order to speed up consciousness. Consciousness is the engine of the mind consisting of electronic representations and through learning, those representations become more complex and through rehearsal, become more accessible, then a higher consciousness is achieved. To put it another way the more control a person has over their environment then the wider the span of consciousness. For instance if a person were left in a dark room, unable to move or sense anything at all then they would be less consciously aware than normal people. Some might argue that the person in the room is just as conscious but in an entirely internal way but what it is in fact, is a lower consciousness because it is not real because consciousness has to be learned. That is why mankind will continue to build and improve on consciousness. Thomas considered the difference in consciousness between the juggler and a person a thousand years from now. The speed could quite possibly be ridiculously fast and that he thought was the way of the world. However, for now Thomas had found his Utopia as he listened to the slight but deep background buzzing of a civilisation at work, like a hive of bees.

Voices from the Ether

It was true to say the middle of the 21st century was a morally and economically turbulent time. Terrorism was the main concern, which was directed at the major democracies that appeared to be excessively decadent in their self obsessed life-styles. The terrorism, which tended to strike anywhere at any time, had the effect it desired. The very foundations of capitalism were no longer looking so strong and freedom was no longer taken for granted in the developed countries. The divide between the haves' and the have-nots was unavoidably increasing. This occurred both within countries and between countries. While the rich owned the factories and machinery to serve industry, the poor had to make do with the menial jobs that insomniac machines were unable to do. Technology fuelling this effect and driving the wedge between the rich and the poor. The poor became small insignificant cogs in big unstoppable wheels. The ideal of a fully automated society was becoming a reality but this western dream was becoming more of a nightmare with so many people becoming unemployed and losing self-esteem and a select few who had it all.

Capitalism seemed decadent and exploited the third world for cheap labour. The third world was doomed for a life in sweat shops being paid a pittance while the fat cats lorded it in the lap of luxury. Even money became a dirty word and any one who had it was put under pressure by journalists to justify themselves and usually they couldn't. A change had occurred. The truth of the matter was that there were no longer any altruistic people working for the good of the world. People were living in cynical times.

Businesses were starting to fail and the economy was taking a major downturn. Many people seemed to be disillusioned about the world including the materialist ideal of capitalism and its opposite, communism with its corruption.

Anyone who was successful tended to be hounded by the press and criticised. They would keep scratching around looking for reasons to put them down and nine times out of ten they would find some scandal behind a person's life and he would then publicly disgraced. The truth of the matter was that completely altruistic businessman or politicians rarely existed anymore and in England, anyone who was successful tended to be looked down upon and the capital ideal was waning.

Then in Japan a minor discovery occurred that would contribute to the shaking of civilisation to the core. A Japanese physicist, Ken Wang, discovered a way to modify radiation. This in itself was no major discovery and proved to have no bounty of applications that so many discoveries have. However, out of mild curiosity he decides to test something that would change his life completely.

He stared at the computer screen that displayed the subtle changes that had been made, and wondered who or what could have made them. What should he do, who should he tell. Ken decides to call on old college friend from Cambridge, Gavin Aldridge.

Gavin flies to Japan after some persuasion from Ken. He steps off the plane and Ken is eagerly waiting for him with his hair unkempt, unshaven and looking like he hasn't slept for a while.

"Hi Gavin, it's good to see you"
"What's all the fuss about Ken, you sounded positively manic on the phone."
"I want to discuss with you a discovery I have made, you're the only qualified person I know to be able to make sense of it."
"Sure but what has my line of work got to do with science."
Ken it seemed had ignored the question.
"Do you think God will ever change the way he works."
"God is always revealing himself to people, he is everywhere, he brings the miracle of life and he performs many other miracles that we are and are not aware of."
"What if someone proves, through science, that he exists?"

"Then I would say he has chosen to reveal himself"

"For what purpose would he want to reveal himself?"

Gavin remains silent; although skeptical he has an element of slight doubt in his mind that Ken was wrong. Ken was a good friend at college and they had many philosophical debates at college. Ken would take a scientific stance and Gavin the opposite. Gavin wondered what fact or discovery was powerful enough for Ken to believe in God and change such a fixed scientific stance.

"We must talk privately back at the lab."

Ken was quiet in the Nissan he was driving from Singapore airport to the science lab on the outskirts he was biting his lower lip. Gavin noticed the streets were full of women demanding equal rights. "Do you get any other marches going on Ken?"

"Oh yes we get the students marching for more subsidies for education, and also we get research companies protesting about certain areas of research being put on hold. It seems the age of achievement is coming to an end, but I hope it's only temporary."

"I'm afraid it's worse in England, we have a yob culture that try to rule the country and woe betide anyone that tries to get in their way. Anyone who is different in any way or anything the yobs don't understand gets hounded out. It all arose from drugs and alcohol. I predicted it years ago when they were becoming the norm. The only way it would end was through infighting. Most of the law-abiding citizens tend to stay indoors now and rarely walk the streets. We live in a culture where cars are the only safe methods of transport but pollute the atmosphere. As for the worlds resources they are getting less available and all we do is print more money, make ourselves richer and decadently materialistic, but increase the world debt. One of these days the whole thing will collapse and then where will we be. I'll tell you stuck on this planet with nowhere to go but to implode. It's the first law of thermodynamics; energy cannot be created nor destroyed. It has to go somewhere and that according to entropy is chaos. We are even finding that the laws of Physics break down at the quantum level, and on it goes."

Ken was silent again and Gavin was deep in thought.

Ken led Gavin out of the car and into his laboratory. It was quite dark and dusty and looked like it needed a spring clean. Not what Gavin had expected at all. Ken waved a hand at all the pizza boxes and mumbled "excuse the mess."

 "So why have you asked me here Ken?"

"I'll start at the very beginning. During the 1960's Physicists were divided and there were two competing theories of cosmology. The Steady State theory, championed by Fred Hoyle and then George Gamow's Big Bang theory. Hoyle and his colleagues maintained that the universe has no beginning or end and that, as the universe expands, matter is spontaneously created to maintain the constant density of the universe.

However, the Big Bang theory was championed by Physicists such as Stephen Hawking and in 1965 an accidental discovery settled the issue."
Ken paused to sip his tea.
"Arno Penzias and Robert Wilson detected a Cosmic Background Radiation. They were looking for signals from the early communications satellites, but they were plagued by background radio noise, corresponding to a temperature of about 3 degrees Kelvin above absolute zero. At first they thought it was white noise caused by pigeon droppings on the satellite dish. They soon realised that the universe was slightly warm or bathed in radiation."

"This is where I come in." said Ken enthusiastically. I discovered that all radiation had a signature and I found it was possible to modify that signature or wavelength."

"So what benefits would that bring? Modifying radiation?" asked Gavin.

"This is so beneficial that our lives rest on it." exclaimed Ken.

"I am sorry, am I missing something Ken."

"I then decided to try and find the Cosmic Background Radiation." Stated Ken with his eyes wide open, as if Simon should understand.
"I set about acquiring the right equipment. I needed a very accurate satellite dish, which took

up most of my savings. It was madness I know but it was a hunch."

"I'm sorry Ken but I'm not getting the big picture here. What has my knowledge or faith in religion got to do with radiation." Gavin studied Christianity at college and now worked for the Church Ministry in England.

"In 2015 I found that the radiation had been changed in some way. I was puzzled at first but then I realised something. Radiation causes mutations in life forms, and so I tested the wavelength and signature of the background radiation. They were exactly right to mutate life and what's more it contained a logical pattern to it." Ken stood up proudly from his seat and concluded, "In my opinion the Cosmic Background Radiation has been steering human evolution. It is possible to read the background radiation because it is not uniform throughout the universe; there are differences or ripples within it. Early scientists believed this was needed to allow the formation of planets and stars. I believe that it goes further by allowing the existence of life forms. The blue print for life is there for all to see. Maybe we were made in Gods eye and maybe the design for life is different in other parts of the universe."

There was one man from the States who made vast amounts of money, honestly. Privately though this man, John Maynard, recognised that the world was waning when it was at its most important phase in its entire history. He perceived that man was currently at its most potentially destructive time and the only way to guarantee its survival was to be living on more than one planet. He felt we were losing our direction at a time when we needed it most. Some leadership was clearly needed but John Maynard didn't have any answers he just knew how to make money. John was helping in the only way he knew how. By investing in two things; the third world and space travel (both commercial and tourism).

John Maynard was beginning to be seen as a cult figure. It was even rumored that he had healing powers but to others this figurehead of capitalism was deeply resented.

As time went on John was becoming more and more resented, by not only his own country but also from other countries. This got so bad that in the end he resorted to growing a beard and dressing down so he wouldn't be recognised. John was soon realising that the money he was investing in developing countries was actually counterproductive. Because the money was given to the people it was often skimmed off through corrupt channels. Often it would end up being used to buy guns for domineering dictators or communist states. It seemed, often, free money didn't work.

After months of real fear John was starting to get seriously worried by the threats he had been receiving. He thought of hiring body guards but felt it would draw attention to him. The shooting of John F. Kennedy had proved that it didn't matter how much protection you had, they could still get to you if they wanted.

Where ever he went he would become self conscious and of course this made it more likely he would be recognised. Even the radio channels were calling for blood. Once, when he was filling his car up with petrol a group of youths approached him. John's heart was pounding in his chest as one of them asked for the time. John naturally looked at his watch and the youth noticed it was a Rolex watch. He looked into John's eyes smiled and pulled out a knife and asked for his wallet and watch. John looked from the youth to the rest of them who were all standing ready. Sweat was beginning to form on his face; if they recognised him he could be facing a problem. John immediately took off his watch and gave it to the boy along with his wallet. Fortunately his wallet contained nothing that would identify him; he had no need for credit cards. The boy looked at the man closely in the eyes; John could see this was a boy with tenacity. John neither prayed nor said anything, his mind was empty and the boys face turned to the side as if trying to perceive something then he blinked, his face returning to its original position but with his chin pulled back a little. The boy slowly backs off keeping his eyes on the businessman; the other boys started jeering the boy, "Go on Strag, cut im." John looks at the other boys most have blood-shot eyes but not all, he looks into Strag's eyes they are sharp and unread. He backs off further and so does John, Strag stops for the briefest of moments and then takes off. John breathes a sigh of relief, seeing the other boys follow their leader.

Simon Percival was busy with his training as a priest, it had been raining a little, while he walked down College Street, but at times the sun shone through. He had been quite a reprobate when he was younger but his father had been strict with him when he was younger and now he was grateful for it, although sometimes he had wished he had a better relationship with his father, one that was perhaps as intuitive as he and his mother's was.

Simon had been to a lecture, which was hailed as one of the most exciting of the year and greatly interested Simon. The subject of the lecture had been "Does the assemblies of God believe that God still performs miracles today?" He found a bench in the university grounds and collected his thoughts; he could see the two sides of the coin. He thought back to the lecture and rewound his Dictaphone to the point where the Priest was summing up… "Assemblies of God believes unequivocally that God still performs miracles today. This conviction grows out of a firm belief that the miracles recorded in the Bible were historical events - not myths or folk stories. There is no indication in scripture that miracles have ceased or will cease in the present world order. Because there are confirmed instances of miracles happening today, we must conclude with certainty that God still performs miracles. Jesus Christ, the greatest worker of miracles is 'the same yesterday, and today, and forever' and that's Hebrews, Chapter13: verse 8. I quote David Hume defining a miracle as 'a violation of the laws of nature'. Faith is an essential element in recognising a miracle. A scientific approach cannot prove or disprove the supernatural validity of a miracle. To the skeptic, such a statement may confirm that miracles do not actually happen, but are real only in the minds of those who choose to believe a miraculous explanation of an event. But the opposite is true. Only the one who believes in the existence of a supernatural God can recognise the hand of God at work. He pauses, as if perceiving something he is unsure of and doesn't know how to react. Simon remembered, he shrugs almost imperceptively and moves on. "However the other danger is the abuse of wanting to help God win the skeptics and impress the saints by describing as miracles certain events which are not divine interventions of God, or by humanly trying to replicate supernatural manifestations of God. God does not need Christians pretending to be miracle workers when God is not the author and the miracle is not genuine. Members of the Assemblies of God must declare always to let God move as He chooses, and never substitute human manifestation for true supernatural miracles. That concludes my lecture, Tha…. Simon turns the machine off.

Gavin engaged Ken in the best way he knew how, carefully. Ken was studying Gavin's face it was quite tranquil then his eyes moved down his body, his arms and hands were open but his toes in his sandals were moving up and down giving away how pensive he was. Gavin asked him "how far are you going to let this go."
"Let what go"
"Well this discovery is your discovery and no-one else's, it belongs to you."
"Exactly when I go public my name will be known as well as Watson and Crick's names were known."
Gavin's lips were pulled back and he took a sharp intake of breath through his teeth. "Are you certain you want to do that Ken?"
"But I'll get the Nobel Peace prize for it."
"Forgive me it is your discovery and I have no business advising you."
"But that's why I asked you here Gav, I want your go ahead on this. I thought you'd be congratulating me."
"The discovery you have made is without doubt the greatest yet. I'm just concerned about how you will manage afterwards."
"Oh sure, I can handle the fame it's just I'm not sure how I'll do on the initial roller-coaster ride

when news breaks. It'll be champagne everywhere and I'll bet I get on the front of Hello magazine."

"It's not that initial stage I'm bothered about. It was a gift to you, from who I'm not sure yet. However, if you depart this gift to the world I'm not sure how it would react to it."

"There'll be dancing in the streets Gav, what are you saying."

" Don't you see," said Gav, his eyes widening fiercely, "If you go public with this discovery, there'll be fighting not dancing"

" I don't understand, you…you…what's the problem with this meeting of science and the Lord God."

"Look Ken you mean well but if you go public with this information, there will be no turning back and the door will be flung wide open. Is that what you want?"

"But we will all believe in God"

"Exactly, if you decide to let the cat out of the bag then we will be taking away other peoples faith, and I'm not sure if we should do that."

" Look Ken that's one of the major parts of religion."

Simon was in a rarely experienced contented mood as he rode his bicycle from the college to his home but that was soon to change. A siren sounded from behind him, a car pulled in from the road and nearly cut Simon's area up. He pulled on the brakes and with his feet lifted his bike onto the pavement and continued to ride on the pavement. Four boys were walking on the pavement and were jeering at a girl they apparently knew on the other side of the street. Simon nearly knocked over one of the boys and he shouted at Simon. Simon continued to persevere with his ride only mildly perturbed. His eyes cast a bit further up the road where he noticed an ambulance was taking off at speed from the street where he lived. He prayed as he cycled, maybe he should have stopped what he was doing and prayed instead but he carried on cycling regardless. He turned a corner to see another ambulance and a police car pulling away. He walked towards where the vehicles had come from and as he got closer he saw a pool of blood on the pavement outside his dormitory house. He walked up to it, noticed its deep red colour. He was mesmerized by it and at that time a boy of around ten years old also walked up to it. They both looked at the blood then into each others faces. Then the boy slowly extended his scuffed shoes and was about to dip his foot into the unsightly pool. Then Simon heard a voice "Don't", he realised the folly and sharply blurted "Don't touch it" to the boy. The schoolboy quickly drew his foot back and walked away without looking at Simon. Simon ran into his bathroom at the end of the corridor, grabbed a bucket and filled it with water. He then washed the pavement of blood, then Prayed in his own way, but as he walked away he noticed some blood was in a footprint shape where he had trodden. He went back to his flat to wash it off and at first thought no more of it.

Months later Simon was at his desk studying hard. He had just read over the last few lines on a document about an individual's personal faith. *In fact*, he thought, *that must be about the tenth time I have read over the past few lines.* Simon's concentration was not as it used to be and his grades had been steadily falling over the past few months. It seemed like the harder he tried the harder it became. After a while he started to doze and it was at this point when he heard a voice calling his name, "Simon". There was no one around and there was none of the usual footsteps in the corridor. There it was again. What seemed to be a voice with power, who was it. God? The devil? He wavered not sure what to do. Then he asked in his mind who is this talking to me. No answer. Eventually he fell back to sleep but in the morning the memory of that voice stayed with him vividly for many years.

At this point in time Ken Wang had decided to go public with his discovery. It made headline news in over thirty of national papers around the globe. He was praised and congratulated and questioned about what he thought it meant. He replied he had no idea. However, one reporter asked him "How are you going to right this terrible wrong - doing you have brought on us." Ken was speechless. "You self righteous reporters cast judgment where you shouldn't. This is a wonderful discovery and I want the world to know it." The reporter spoke under his breath inaudibly "Merde." It was not quite picked up by Ken but he knew something was uttered and he guessed it was negative.

People started speculating what this discovery would mean. The scientists were exploring the fact that if there are aliens out there then maybe they would look like us, provided, they said, that the background radiation is uniformed throughout the universe. There were many new experiments being designed hastily to replicate the experiment and at the same time many spin off experiments.

The theologians were arguing amongst themselves and it almost broke some arms of organised Religion apart, trying to explain the findings in a divine way. There were some schools of thought that said Armageddon was upon us, others said it was the second coming, and others said God was telling us to cool off and think about what we were doing. Many religious cults sprang up, one, quite widespread over a period of time, said that aliens similar to ourselves who had religion the same as ours, with a Son of God and an Adam and Eve, and were out there in the same position as us. Perhaps there were many pockets of humans out there. However, this was not the mainstream view and most did not believe that others were trying to contact us.

Simon could see that society started to break down once again. This time Simon was unsure why. With proof that God existed, Simon couldn't understand why this was happening. Simon wasn't sure all he knew was that society was breaking down and something needed to be done about it. How this happened, people were unsure.

A few days later he received his answer in the form of a voice in his head while he was driving in his newly acquired car. *Simon you need to ask Jesus.* It seemed plain to Simon that this was God talking to him, but what did he mean. How can he go to Jesus? How can he travel back?

Over the next few months Simon could see society breaking down before his very eyes and was anxious to do the right thing. Except he didn't know what that was. He did his best to follow the voices but he wasn't sure what they were telling him. Some seemed to tell him one thing and others another. Some commented on what he was thinking others inserted thoughts into his head. Sometimes he would find he had thought blocks, thoughts he couldn't get past. Other times his thoughts would snag on something that he couldn't get out of his mind. Sometimes he heard good voices like his brother encouraging him on. However, after a great deal of time had passed Simon was still fighting with his voices and it seemed he was no closer to his goal. How can he go back in time when it seemed we were a long way away from time travel technology.

As time went on Simon's voices came and went, came and went. Sometimes he managed to enjoy life quite well, but he always returned to his delusions in a kind of love hate sort of way. He was in some way tied to them, like a moth to the moon. At the same time Simon was determined to continue with his Theology degree, which although hard he was determined to succeed at. It was strange really he could not let go of his delusions or of trying to succeed in the real world. The question of deciding which he wanted never occurred to him and he was luckily never asked to decide between the two. So he stuck by both through thick and thin. Sometimes his delusions would get the better of him and he was unable to go on placement or to college and other times he was engrossed in his college work and able to ignore the voices.

As time went on he began to get messages from the TV and radio. Still he would not let go of the fact that "God" had spoken to him and at the same time let go of his career. He felt special but still wanted to do well as an ordinary person.

Then after a time his voices were getting more and fiercer "God" seemed more demanding and the "devil" seemed plain petrifying. But still he persisted. He started reading papers and tried to ignore the messages he was getting and then he read about John Maynard. "God" told him that John was similar to himself and that he must contact him. This he did in person. He tracked John down in America and went to see him.

After some deft persuasion, as mad people can often do, John agreed to see him. Simon walked into his office and felt the sumptuous carpet beneath his feet. He was going to comment on it but decided not to. John similarly looked guarded. "I've come to give you a message." John looked across the desk at him "oh what is that?" "You and I have been chosen to visit Jesus and gain knowledge from him on how to run the planet, at this crucial time."

The talking went on for a long time with differing results. John thought he was a nut and Simon thought he was getting through to John. Making progress, it was easier than he thought. However, John was a sensible man and realising this meant he was on a completely different path and thus merely agreed with him. He knew something needed to be done but Simon's proposal was too outlandish.

Simon, on returning home started reading the paper for a third person. He took a guess that it could be someone from Japan, but he wasn't sure. Meanwhile his fears and visions were getting stronger and when he closed his eyes at night he could see flashes of different scenes. It was as if he was looking at a television and someone was changing channels really fast. He also heard news items, in his head, mentioning his name.

After every episode he had he would at some point come back and get what he called "the flip". This was a point at which he would gain insight into what he was now beginning to believe was a mental illness.

However.

Simon kept pushing his delusions and sad to say that at some points his delusions (which he usually kept on his left) and reality (which he usually kept on his right) had started to merge once again. Instead of just a matter of a couple of weeks these delusions were lasting longer and had never been so real.

At this time his psychiatrist had put him on a new drug. This had a paradoxical effect. Firstly it made the voices more powerful but also armed him with the energy to deal with the voices. By this time he had learned not to interact with them or answer back or give any sort of opinion what-so-ever. He still wasn't sure if he was delusional or that there was truth in it. He could feel the power of the voices was waning and he felt he was making progress.

Over time Simon found he could communicate with other people around him and one day he found his mind could cast to any-ware and anyone in the world; Prime-ministers, presidents, despots, dictators and enemies of the civilized world. He felt if he only listened to people in his mind he could prevent death and destruction. He could feel all the millions of minds meshing with his and then a wonderful but deeply terrifying silence......, then a small but definite sound. It was a single lone gunshot going off, from the West's side of troops at war, he could tell. It made him jump and immediately shouted "NO, no shooting!" It went dead back to an even more terrifying silence. He hesitated not knowing what to do and in that instant the other side started firing back then gunfire from both sides rising to a crescendo of death and destruction. This proved to Simon that he was unable to sort the world's problems out quite so easily.

God had told him that the person he needed to see was the Japanese scientist Ken Wang, whom he had heard about from his discovery of Gods blue print for the human race present in the cosmic background radiation. He could not afford to fly out to the scientist's home in Japan so he sent him a letter telling Mr. Wang that he had been chosen by God to somehow go back to see Jesus and gain wisdom from his teachings and to be able to overcome society's problems.

Simon received no reply or correspondence from either Maynard or Wang until the summer when on a hot sultry day he was laying on the grass in the garden of his rented accommodation and he heard someone trying to contact him. He knew because he had a wonderful head rush and John Maynard said "I'm in". He then thought he heard Ken Wang say something but he couldn't be sure. He didn't get the head rush so he thought Japan wasn't in. This he thought was logical because of that country's past. They once believed their emperor was a God and perhaps thought they couldn't commit to this new and radical plan.

So it was that Simon Percival and so he believed John Maynard embarked on a mission to bring world peace.

Simon had already found he could communicate with the past through television and radio and he felt the difficult part would be avoiding King Herod as it said in the Bible.

Simon was again lying in his garden when his mind started turning to Jesus. He could feel his mind and John Maynard's too (or what he thought was Maynard. He ,still, was not sure if Maynard went along with what he said, to this day) gradually going back through history and he knew the world was listening in. He pulled his thoughts back and prayed to God then tentatively started to push through the ages. Through the world wars then the Renaissance then Medieval times (this he found difficult getting through but he coped) then to the days of the Roman Empire and finally to Jesus. He took a tentative mental step towards the Lord Jesus then Jesus exclaimed 'wait for me here"
And so it was that Simon Percival went down in history as making the biggest mistake ever.
Nobody knew who Simon was or what he looked like but nearly everyone saw a little of what he had done and every so often someone might see him

and wonder if it was him. Some smiled and some cursed, but he still wasn't sure what he did wrong.

Then one day Simon heard a short firm knock at the door. He dragged himself off the sofa and pushed his hair back from his face.
It was Ken Wang.
 "Are you Simon Percival?"
"Yes"
"The same Simon Percival who wrote this letter to me"
"Yes that's me"
"Can I come in Mr. Percival"
"Yes of course, I would offer you some tea but I'm out of teabags" Simon replied whilst at the same time cautiously shutting the door behind him.
"I've come to try to right a terrible wrong that I did."
"I thought I was the only one to make terrible mistakes."
"Oh I doubt that very much." Said Ken
"Do you know where you went wrong Simon"
"No it felt … necessary."
"Maybe it was a question of faith or lack of it. I mean why didn't you have faith in God to help us out of life's problems."
"Yes I see that now"
"But you still don't see quite where you went wrong"
"Life is about the struggle. We can't just expect God to get us out of our problems."
"Oh" sniffed Simon

"You forget that Jesus is here, in our hearts. He is all around us and he's up there" Simon's eyes opened wide in recognition.

"You can talk to him at anytime. You don't have to play silly mind games to hear his way. I am certain that God talks in feelings and emotions and not through voices"

The End

Widows Peak

Sometime just before the swarm centuries, an obscure scientist, Richard Jenkins is in the Arizona Sonora Desert in search of a handful of pre-selected animals that live in this inhospitable habitat. This man has scoured two thirds of the globe, mostly in extreme environments, as these, he thinks, will produce what he is looking for. The sun's increased energy speeds up these animals' metabolisms, enhancing any advantages they may have. He is in search of something that may not even exist. What is he studying? Some say he is a nut, others deny he is a scientist, but what counts is what he believes. He is studying Para-biology or at least trying to create it in humans from animals. No-one knows if humans had any undiscovered mental abilities in their past, perhaps before they had language but not now. Richard Jenkins knows this because he has developed a machine to test this and he has tested humans and found nothing.

That's why he has turned to animals to test them for possible mental powers. He knows not what to expect but if he is successful he knows exactly what to do with them, what he wasn't aware of was the forces he would unleash.

His guide lifted a stone and out scurried a scorpion. It scampered across the scientist's boot. He jumped back a few feet and the guide, Dave, started laughing, picked the scorpion up by its tail and held it out for the scientist to '*test it for God knows what*' he thought. Jenkins, sweating, grunted and wiped his face. He wasn't keen on creepy crawlies but his projections predicted one of the highest possibilities for finding what he was looking for. This time though, as was the case so many thousand times before, he detected nothing. He looked up at the sky, shielding his eyes from the sun and thought maybe the spiders "yes the spiders" he muttered. "Spiders, did you say" the guide pointed to an oasis in the valley. Dave walked and Richard trudged on towards a place the guide often thought of as magical. It had entered his dreams many times and he had been visiting this place since he was a child.

Jenkins had tested so many thousands of species in the past. He had noticed that when birds fly in flocks they would all turn at the same time and he wondered if they had telepathic abilities. Similarly he tested fish because of the way they swam in shoals. He tested fire flies because their abdomens flashed altogether in unison across dozens of the flashing fly laden trees at a time. He tested the duck-billed platypus which, he learned, could seek out its prey by sensing an animal's electrical currents in its nerves, with its duck bill. These creatures were of interest for another reason. As human females have an xx chromosome and the males an xy, the platypus females have five xx chromosomes and the males five xy. This information could have pointed the way to the possibility of psychic ability. But alas all lacked mental powers.

If it hadn't been for Richard Jenkins diligence, commitment, and determination then maybe mankind's dark future could have been avoided, but this was not the first time the world would have to pay for a scientist thinking he had a bright idea and it probably wouldn't be the last.

Maybe the brain is a universe in itself and thoughts are living things which thrive or die according to natural laws. Maybe synapses were at one time cellular organisms that lived in symbiosis in the brain and competed to survive. Just as mitochondria, a cells energy source, are thought to have been once cellular organisms that were symbiotic and as a result gave humans advantages for advantages to themselves in return. The result was assimilation by the body.

Whatever the theory the fact remained that this scientist had an idea and he felt it should be tested as to whether or not it actually existed.

The fact that this idea caste shadows was neither here nor there according to Richard Jenkins. In fact, he may have known this on a subconscious level but a scientist being a man of logic, of black and white perceptions, his ken was skewed and unable to foresee basic complications in his plans. In practice, the idea seemed to perpetuate itself, a life of its own. What force that gave it this momentum is still to this day unknown.

His guide trudged on ignoring the scientists' grunts and groans about the speed of their journey. At last they came to the trees and shrubs. The guide walked through the undergrowth and stopped at a small fallen tree that he said was gradually being decomposed by many life forms and would be a haven for a whole host of critters he could test.

Richard spots something that the guide hasn't. His eyes light up and points to the animal and asks him what species is it. "Yes, that's the Black Widow, a female I think." "Just the sex I'm looking for, in this species anyway." He lowers the instrument to the spider. As with most scientists he was mildly euphoric when he smelt the possibility of success, as if the feeling was a drug. His pack, with the universal energy amplifier, starts to crackle, he adjusts the filter controls and then it bleeps, once at first then in quick succession, he shouts "well, guide, I have just found the biological equivalent of gold". And so it was that Richard Jenkins, the scientist, thought of as a bit of a nut, was vindicated at last. However, as things are never as good or as bad as they seem, there was a flipside to the discovery. Just as Jenkins takes his instrument away the spider leaps towards it and just nicks the man's hand. The guide swears at him "I told you not to get too close to the venomous types". The scientist, not realizing the seriousness of his error exclaims "Oh

I'll be alright. It was just a nip" and rubs his hand. The guide immediately grabs his hand and puts it in his mouth biting around the spiders bite. "Ow, that hurts!" "Look, what would you prefer" says the guide "to die or lose a small piece of flesh". The Scientist still only mildly perturbed and still not realizing the seriousness of this event sniffs and holds his hand out and turns his face away. The guide bites and sucks at the flesh and puts a tourniquet around his wrist. "Come, we must hurry."

The hospital was 2 hours drive away and they have to walk over a kilometer to the land rover. The guide is faced with a dilemma, make him run to the vehicle, or walk and prevent his body carrying the venom round it. Already the skin on his hand is starting to darken and the guide is worried. The guide having always been careful of the land and its laws of nature had never been bitten or had to deal with another person having a venomous bite. The guide tries to remember his training, which was years ago. Jenkins is oblivious to all this and is ranting about how he will receive the Nobel Peace prize. Soon the pain spreads to his arm and Jenkins begins to worry a little when he notices the guide looking anxiously at the spread of the Black Widows potentially fatal venom. Jenkins starts to flag at this point and asks for a rest to catch his breath. The guide denies him. The car is still not in sight and the guide is talking to Richard to keep him conscious while he now carries him. "So what were you testing for back there, my friend?"

"Psionics" he rasps." Tell me about it." Jenkins thinks about it and looks around as if not knowing where he is. "I was testing for ESP and I have found it exists in that little spider of yours."

"And what will you do with this discovery of yours?"

"I…..sequence the…….insert……!"

The guide assumes the man is delusional and makes a final push for the land rover.

In the four by four, the guide looks over at Jenkins who is in a fitful sleep and he sees the torment on the eccentric man's face. Jenkins drifts through visions of spiders crawling towards him. Then the scene changes and he sees televisions being changed channels in quick succession, all are visions of death and destruction. Then suddenly he looks down at himself and spiders are crawling all over him. He screams and the guide puts a hand to his forehead to calm him and check his temperature. The man was burning up. The guide steps up the speed on his land rover, "this won't do my suspension any good" and he stifles a curse from escaping from his mouth for letting Jenkins get so close to the spider.

Richard Jenkins was, after nearly two and a half hours, elsewhere in his mind. Where, no-one could say, except for those that had experienced a venomous bite before. Maybe he was drifting between this world and the next, but whatever; the guide could see he was beginning to lose him.

"Just minutes longer" encouraged the guide. They were within sight of the hospital, and then suddenly Jenkins sat up, his eyes wide open, as if in a moment of great clarity and asked the guide "Dave?"

"Yes Richard"

"I'm not a bad person, am I". The guide looks deep into his eyes and exclaims in a wise but sad way "No Richard, you are not a bad man; in what little time I've known you!"

The spider's psionics seem to be a coercion field, which according to a battery of tests allows the spider to catch (by coercing them into its web) insects.

With an inevitable explosion in genetics that rivals the technological revolution, it was made possible under the guidance of the recovered Jenkins to sequence the spider's psi gene and transplant it into human DNA.

The first humans to have the genes were normal in every way except they were said to be charismatic. However, as the generations grew and died and selective breeding in this area became commonplace people became better and better at this coercion. The advantages to this special ability were immediately obvious and many people wanted the gene.

However at one point in time, the psi ability was disallowed because free will was thought to have been eroded by its use. The coercers were forbidden to breed in order to prevent any possible oppression, but that just sent the coercers underground or to countries that didn't prevent it. As a result of this these people learned to hide their ability, only using it rarely and subtly but by the time people realized it truly darkened Homosapiens' potential it was too late.

The decision was later reversed, mainly because the most influential people at that time were exactly that, the most influential. They were all mostly coercers. The phenomena had gone too far to stop. For better or worse, Man, it seemed was changed forever.

The future wasn't all doom and gloom though; in fact it was because it was so prosperous that people largely disregarded the coercion gene. As long as the profits kept rolling in from the work of machines then the majority were happy. This majority spent most of their time designing a vast array of machines to do more and more varied tasks and then machines to build those machines. Machines were being used in every thing including the computer arts and ever outlandish leisure pursuits. Computers were blurring the edges of reality and fantasy. The middle classes tended to be careful to try and control their offspring to stop their immersion in to fantasy that computers fuelled and to do their best to keep the two separate. For children to learn what counts in life and what doesn't so much in the myriad of fantasy contortions and contusions. But humanity was moving closer to a fully automated society.

The next few centuries, despite this worrying form of mental power that some had, was a time of great discovery, expansion and glory both in science and space travel. Society becoming virtually fully automated, this augmented space travel and made it especially fruitful. In fact fruitful was a good word for it, as the ships that went through space provided the seeds to colonize other planets. They were known as Von Neumann probes. These were self-replicating machines, specifically designed for space exploration and colonization. It was named after John Von Neumann (1903-1957), a Hungarian-born American mathematician and physicist who specialized in the field of self-replicating machines.

These probes would be launched to a neighboring star-system. Upon its arrival it would immediately seek out raw materials on asteroids, moons, or gas giants to create replicas of itself. Once it had created a sufficient number of replica probes, the original probe to enter the system went about exploring that star-system.

These probes were sent out with a number of items on board. Firstly, they contained within them nanotechnology. These would terraform the chosen habitat to human requirements. They were also sent with fertilized human embryos which were artificially born when the habitat was ready to be colonized. Also on board the ship were several androids, whose purpose it was to nurse and teach the young humans to the best of their abilities. Communication was used between planets so as to keep the community with as many human traits as possible. A number of computer terminals were on board which not only contained a line to the rest of the human race (for which life was becoming exactly that, a race) but also a database with as much knowledge, facts and even legends that were possible.

At first the probes were designed to build habitats rather than terraform planets, like the Stanford Torus,

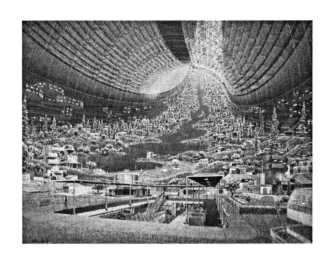

O'Neill Cylinder

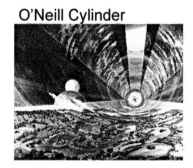

Bernal Sphere

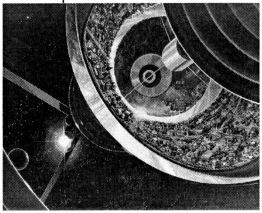

And eventually Dyson Spheres, a habitat built around a small star.

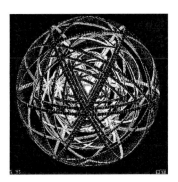

Later the probes were sent deeper into space to find suitable planets and moons to terraform. The Von Neumann probes were like futuristic Noah's Arks.

Von Neuman probes were sent out further and further a field.

After several centuries of this expansion and proliferation of man, there was an unfortunate side effect. It became known as the "Brutality of Capitalism" or "Resource Drain". It was the simple effect of humans' materialistic ways which led to a drought of resources in the centre of man's territory. This occurred on the oldest inhabited planets. At first technology utilized resources and energy more frugally but sadly it could not match the marching spread of humans throughout the galaxy. People were horrified to learn in schools that historically oil and coal and wood were burnt just to keep people warm. It was an unfortunate effect of mans' so called civilization that left many people, on the central planets, too poor to buy passage to greener pastures. The situation was a negative feedback cycle. As resources became scarcer it got harder to send ships to the fringe, where life flourished. Even the weather was fought over for crucial rain fall. Countries fight for rainwater by seeding clouds with silver iodide crystals to make them rain on their territory. Yet another way the rich could use money to squeeze a planet literally dry.

As a result of this lack of resources, transport became more expensive and fewer inhabitants could afford to travel. This resulted in a slow moving shock wave that started slowly and speeded up. It was dependent on the technology of travel and money itself. Only the rich stay at the periphery, or the cusp of life. It had a whole new effect on the value of money. It seemed that capitalism was fuelling a new form of survival of the fittest which in itself led to an exodus of the rich. Once again the poor suffered.

There was a number of ways that the poorer planets tried to remedy this. The most successful curbing of capitalist ways which among other things occurred in supermarkets. The store cards people were issued with, analysed a person's wealth by what they bought and how extravagant they were when spending money, the more extravagant the more they were charged. The product "wants" were more money than the "needs". Alas the efforts made buy big companies was not enough to prevent the explosion of degradation.

Some of the poor people saved some money to be put into cryogenic sleep. Others simply stopped having children and faded away. There were also fewer charities for the poor as the rich clung on to their savings to guarantee their own privileged position and to guarantee the survival of their genes via their offspring. The poor lay in stasis on ships trying to get to a safer land hoping to be revived by others. As was so often the case, if there wasn't any money in this then it was in vain. The very poor died. Little did they know that in the eyes of some, they were the lucky ones?

As the generations came and went it became more and more desirable to have the coercive ability discovered by Jenkins, and of course the strongest were the most successful.

Eventually it became a leadership contest between master coercers. With each generation, the strongest became the emperor. When an emperor became so charismatic, and it was believed that eventually one would, then he would be able to command the majority of all humans to do anything he liked, including fight. This person would be known as the Widower and would be greatly feared by the people.

Seven centuries after the scientist Jenkins idea, life in the human sector of the universe was very different from what it was then.

The advisor opened the huge door to the palace as he had done so many times before but this time he was hit by the immense decadence of the building. A show of power of the man whom he would soon be up against. He was beginning to see the Widower for what he really was, a man who said all the right things, but cared little for his fellow man. Fortunately for the Widower he no longer needed to coerce people much now. The human race knew he could bend a majority of their minds to his will and the prize for their forced allegiance was a free ticket to his apparent paradise.

The Colonel was dreading giving the news.

His knees were losing their effectiveness as the thoughts of what he was about to report began to grate on his mind, and soon his mind would grate a whole lot more if the Emperor had anything to do with it.

He opened the door to the Emperor's chamber and fell to his knees, "maybe he'll go easy" he thought, but he knew it was a desperate situation. "What news, do you bring, Colonel?" The Officer replies, "We still have not found the resistance's outpost, Emperor, however, we are searching and have limited it down to a handful of locations."

The situation was not as straight forward as it seems. The Emperor, although outwardly tyrannical in his approach to others, was actually in himself a reserved man with a conscience. However, as with any visionary, he was required to stamp his authority on the Empire in order to bring that vision to life. That vision was so crucial to him that his ends justified his means. The sad truth was that this vision was both single-minded and clouded by his off kilter sense of right and wrong. He felt that to do any good in the world he had to bring about change which required the use of force for his dream to be a reality. His sight remained targeted on one thing and one thing only - Omnipotence and his place at its head. The Widower knew he was close to realizing his ambition of a new era.

The Widower turns to look at the Colonel. He holds the Colonel's eye contact a little longer than was comfortable for the Colonel who moves his weight from right foot to left.

"There have been reports of a large number of ships heading for the planet Metarhar. I want you to comb that planet for the last resistance outpost."

Meanwhile a grim faced mother is pushing her way through the market in a war torn city, on a greatly diminished planet as was the case with a sizeable proportion of habitable land at mankind's poor self defeated nucleus these days. The war between the Old and the New Church saw to that. Her eyes are flitting from one stall to the next, avoiding the watchful gazes of the similarly poor stall holders who have to pay absorbitant prices to display their wares. She lives on a world called Titan which is not far from Ganymede, they both orbit Saturn.

She has in tow a daughter named Lydia who is helping her spot any opportunities. The mother has to feed the girl and she gently pulls on her arm to draw her attention, then her other hand goes out to grab a swamp tuber, the stall owner sees the hand and immediately stops bartering with a tall pasty looking man and shouts "Stop, thief!"

The woman runs and Lydia follows. She knows when to do this as they have done it many times before. Lydia's mother had to steal food to live. If it was because she didn't know how to earn a living, it was because she was never shown. If she did know of an alternative way of living, it was unattainable. No one knew this woman's dreams, or aspirations that she may have had when she was young because she had never shared them with anyone and now it was just a desperate situation. She lived day to day caring for her only family, her daughter. She knows the stall holders usually don't give chase, but she knows the Bots may be watching. Even on this world so far away from the edge some Bots remain to maintain order. She was unaware of the robots presence so near to her. The tall pasty man shrugs off his cloak and Lydia catches a glimpse of a weapon emerging from his arm and slipping into his hand. The man is not human but a Bot, something to be feared because of their ruthlessness. Lydia shouts "A Bot!" and they push on faster as they hear the Bot issue its warning in the name of the Emperor. The Bot begins to run holding the sonic gun deadly straight. It's taking long effective strides and is closing the gap. The mother tells Lydia "split." They know now what to do even though this has never happened before. The mother was thoughtful in her plans. The two change directions. Lydia's heart is in her throat, she secretly hopes the Bot will follow her but suspects it'll go for her mother because she stole the tuber. She risks a glance behind her and she does a double take. There was no one following or within discernable sight. The crowd seems to have swallowed them both up. She stops, slightly breathless, and retraces her steps and reaches the crowd. There is a closeness in the air that hints fog is on its way. An animal slinks in front of her, but her legs single mindedly walk forward mimicking the Robot she is trying to track, the animal squeaks and hops away. She knows the Robot's mind is centrally controlled.

The girl, Lydia, never sees her mother in the crowd. She searches for three days but to no avail. She did think she heard her mother calling her name but when she turned, her heart jumping- she scanned the area from the market to the horizon for many minutes, how long she knew not, her heart sank as she supposed it must have been the wind.

After searching she lumbered home utterly dejected and slumped in her mother's favorite chair. Exhausted, her mind on a level so low she had never experienced and in her stupor she hoped never to feel this way again. She scanned the room and took all the sensations in, seeing it from a different viewpoint. The Russian doll on the mantelpiece, the Titan Angel next to it. She remembers her father telling her about the Angel and that when Titan was first colonized the atmosphere was so thick and gravity so low that its inhabitants could don wings and fly. She looks down at her toys on the floor and they no longer seem of any use. There was no sound in the room at all, she was exhausted and she felt like she was cocooned in a state between sleep and daydreaming. The clock on the wall was silent which bought pain inside her stomach, time seemed shored up. She looked back to the flowers then at the Titan figurine and crossed her fingers as a cold shiver went down her spine. She then looked curiously at the picture of her grandfather and grandmother. Lydia sat looking out of the window for some hours watching the birds and other animals eating the last of the stale bread that had been put out by her mother, before what was known by Psychiatrists as Lydia's Primary Event (The loss of her mother - the last of her remaining family). This Primary Event would define her choice of future decisions and actions. She pinches the top of her nose screws her fists into the wells of her eyes and forcefully rubs them. Her hands move together and she pinches the flesh between thumb and index finger on both hands. Her eyes flicker in random directions; she feels cold and senses an instant of hope that she will feel better in the morning. She then faltered as if by a lack of faith due to a reassessment and found she was reluctant to sleep…

She was reluctant to sleep because when she woke she knew that her situation would seem all the more real. As though it would seal her mother's fate. Her exhaustion hit her like a wave but she sensed some intelligence flit in and out of her consciousness. It lay beyond reach but she sensed it and that was enough.

The next morning when the last of the bread was taken she had a little cry and finally felt a little release. She pulled herself together as best she could, then felt she had better get her affairs in order as she knew the authorities would be coming. She went into the study to look through all her mother's papers. She spent some time looking through some bills and then her attention wandered, whereabouts she wasn't sure but her eyes fell on a book called the family bible. She pulled this, the largest of the books, from the shelves and carefully opened the first page. Inside were two things. A leaflet titled 'Omega-the Church of the Modern Era' and also her family tree in her fathers hand.

She sat on the chair and pulled the bible closer. She noticed that the family tree went back nine centuries. Then her eyes fell on the name Jenkins seven centuries before her name. Jenkins rang a bell so she consulted her computer. Her heart sank as she accessed Richard Jenkins profile inside her internal computer in her stomach. Her ancestor Richard Jenkins was the man who was responsible for coercion and had unwittingly produced the Widower. She buries her face in her hands at the thought of this news. Lydia then puts the leaflet in her pocket.

Curious she reads on in this strange book with its mysterious pictures and finds it is a book about a man named Christ. This man gave rise to a religion called Christianity. She looks up the word Christianity. No hits. She looks up Christ. No hits again. She vaguely remembers her mother mentioning a good man named Jesus Christ but that's all she knew.

Just then her ring buzzes so she answers the call and on the line is a very faint sound. She listens intently and the sound seems pleasant so she listens a little more and the sound, continuing to hold her attention, made her intensely curious on a subliminal level. At this time two things happened, firstly she saw movement from the corner of her eye through the window and then she heard the melody draw nearer to her head. It was strange but intriguing. In the instant when she could feel it about to pervade her very spirit, her attention was faintly drawn to the movement and this was just enough to allow her to drag her ear away from the phone. Some music, Lydia knew, could induce some basic emotions and can be a powerful tool to those with knowledge of it.

And so she was able to hang up the phone and shake her head clear. The four men were approaching the house and she noticed two of the men walk round towards the back of the house and so she climbed out of the window and ran east towards the war torn city. She swore to herself knowing that the world was so riddled with war, so much so that she could not scrape a living and must avoid the authorities at all cost. She knew little about the reasons for war except to say that she did not believe the Widower's intensions were honorable. This she learned from her grandfather who taught her how to read a person's face and speech patterns. The widower, she knew, spoke passionately but showed little anxiety or care for sending his men to war against the resistance. She never heard anything positive of the resistance in the media. Lydia was unaware that an artificial intelligence had been controlling the information highways and building a large propaganda machine in favor of the New Church. Also, Lydia did not know that soon she would experience the power of the Widower directly for herself.

She found refuge under a bypass road and finally fell into a deep dreamless sleep.

She was woken by some tramps nearby singing as they drank alcohol. Lydia watched them as they drank like babies sucking a bib.
She stretched her arms then rubbed her hands to warm them, and then put them in her coat pockets. She felt the leaflet that had been found inside the Bible.
She read it from beginning to end. She had seen many similar leaflets beforehand but on this one there was a line written in her father's hand. Her father had died just four and a half years after she was born. How she didn't know.

Omega-The Church of the Modern Era

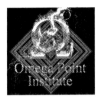

Dear Friend,

"Before you throw out the old ways, you must have something of value with which to replace them."

The wisdom of this ancient Kikuyu saying is being borne out all over mans domain today. Have you noticed the evil operating in the many worlds but are amazed that our popular culture is blind to it and helpless before it?

Have you noticed how much of this evil is perpetrated in the name of fragmented religions and cults?
Are you someone whose scientific education and/or knowledge of the bloody histories of the

major religions prevent you from enjoying the moral certitude that believers have always lived in?

I invite you to join in the most important adventure of the new era. Help us create a church that is integral with scientific thought, not embarrassed by it, yet provides a solid moral grounding, a ground of being that will truly save, nourish and heal our species.

Have you noticed the moral poverty and confusion of our society? Do you believe Evil exists, yet no one is talking about it, much less fighting it?

Isn't it time to replace your allegiance to transient and ineffective religions with allegiance to our whole species? Our species is at risk, what are you doing about it?

Do any of these thoughts resonate with you? Then please help us. Now is the time for you to be a Cofounder of The Church of the Modern Era.

Thinkers of our Worlds unite! You have nothing to lose but your confusion; you have a Universe to gain.

Sincerely,

The universe is a womb for the genesis of gods.

The Way of the Cosmic Chain of Being of
The Church of the Modern Era

Beliefs:

There is a Cosmic Chain of Being that runs from
the beginning of time in our Universe through the
stars, the planets, blue green algae, the early
hominids, the first Homo-Sapiens, Confucius,
Moses,
Aristotle, Socrates, Plato, Galileo, Newton, Darwin,
Einstein, our ancestors, us, our descendents and
successors to God.

We have developed an understanding and control
of biology; matter and energy; time and space;
technology. There is Good and Evil in this
Universe and we must see that Good triumphs in
the God Time and not Evil.

God can bring us back to life and reunite us with
our loved ones in Virtual Heaven, Hell or
Purgatory. We must see that this happens.

As ancestors and children of God, it is our First
Sacred Duty to defeat Evil and perfect ourselves,
our families and our species to be worthy of this
gift and to wisely guide the Cosmic Chain of Being.

We are all equal before God, but we are each
unique.

Follow the Church of the new era and your future in virtual heaven will be guaranteed. Stand in our way and you risk either oblivion or virtual hell.

Heresy

The last word was written in her father's handwriting.

She thought about the war between the new and the old churches. She wasn't sure what each of the Churches stood for. Only that the Widower was a bad person. Her mother always taught her to respect tradition and her school teachers were required to teach Lydia of the benefits of technology and that it would provide mans' salvation. Her teachers always taught this sort of information in a flat monotone voice and sometimes Lydia wondered why they said such flattering words for the New Church, she was very confused. Her mind flicked back to a time when her mother taught her about a legend of a man named Christ, whom she had read about the day before. This man gave his life in order to found a Religion with God. It was called Christianity.

Lydia was slowly and aimlessly walking down a street towards the park. She cared not where her feet took her as her mind was focused on the digital information being sent from her abdomen.

When anyone is born in the Empire they are genetically altered before birth and the result of this is a baby with three arms. The third arm grows from the chest and some time after birth, these babies undergo an operation whereby all the flesh and bone of the arm gets stripped away and the remaining nerves get attached to a bio-computer that is firstly linked to the net and secondly gains nourishment from the body's energy and so grows as the child grows. The computer is put in the child's stomach. Nerves interacting with silicone. Some call it a Symbiont but a few people, like her grandfather, warned her not to rely on its security. Why, Lydia was unsure.

When scientists were looking for ways to interface computers with the brain they realized that the brain cerebrum was too vast and complex and too individualistic to allow for a direct form of interaction to be possible. As a result the nerves and the computer were put inside the belly. Children generally mastered using this by around six years, often just after they learned to read. What she doesn't know is that also when she looked up the term Christianity in her body's computer, all information is monitored and if necessary, passed to the Widower.

The lack of information on this subject puzzled Lydia as there should be some information regarding this religion. She had found similarly no evidence other Religions of similar times. The knowledge about this man had come from two sources so she couldn't understand why the net didn't have any information about it. The net she knew still had some quite ancient sites that were now protected by heritage organizations.

Lydia was beginning to distinguish the lies and the truth.

By now, a vast computer, which the Widower was in direct contact with, was alerted to Lydia's enquiry and managed to get a position lock on her. The computer then alerted the Widower and gave her position to him.

Lydia got up feeling a bit lost and helpless so she went to the park. She couldn't go home as the authorities would be waiting for her and she wasn't sure what they would do to someone without any support from relatives. She was right to fear them. The law was no longer about justice but more about subduing outbreaks of unrest in a long forgotten and stagnant part of mans' domain. She reached the park and it was overgrown in most areas, however as she walked she came across an old haggard gentleman whom she assumed was the park gardener because he was tending to a small oasis garden. He looked up at her with a large bulbous nose, bags under his eyes, a stooped back and a black and white border collie that started sniffing round her feet. The man called the dog, "Spot", back to his side and continued with his gardening. He nodded to Lydia and moved away from the entrance to tend to a white rose. This allowed Lydia to walk into the garden and at the back of the garden she saw a bench which she wished to sit on to draw on the serenity of this oasis. So she walked round the garden towards it. She looked at the flowers as she went, there were herbs of all different sorts. She picked a leaf at random while the man wasn't looking and rubbed the leaf bringing it to her nose. The smell reminded her of a memory from a long time ago, when, she wasn't sure but it included her family. She held the leaf and walked on and she got a brief but strong smell of lavender as she neared the bench. This was her grandfather's and his father's favorite smell. She wiped the dew off the bench with her handkerchief and carefully sat down on the bench, aware only of herself and the few feet around her. The light seemed to darken slightly and she felt downcast, her head lowered. She saw a stick on the floor and so she picked it up and pulled out her pocket knife to begin whittling it unsure of what to make out of it. Then a strange feeling came over her, whom she disliked so she started to sharpen the stick and with each stroke of the knife her mood darkened. Then suddenly she felt a sharp compulsion to stab herself in her chest. The shear force of this urge surprised her and made her fearful. The feeling grew stronger so she dropped the sharpened wood and then tried to drop the knife but her grip only tightened around it. It was as if this thought had been inserted into her mind and it seemed to overpower her love even for her own mother. She hated herself for this and the compulsion grew stronger, it was then she realized that whatever this force was she must fight it for her very survival.

Lydia's survival instinct was very strong but her hand was held stark still with the knife over her chest. It was drawing close to the centre of her chest and it penetrated slightly and where it nicked was the scar tissue where her arm had been stripped of flesh after her birth. The old man muttered the word "computer". She suddenly remembered her bio-computer and it was enough to make a connection between the computer and this urge. So she pulled the knife towards her belly and stabbed herself. She pulled the knife carefully but forcefully down. The pain was excruciating and she would not have been able to continue had she not felt the soothing power from the gardener and so she could reach in and grab the pulsating computer. She quickly severed the nerves as she screamed. The pain was still burning through her head pulsing through her it was like cutting off her hand. The gardener came running and put his shirt over the gape in her belly and took her to his car (a rare thing on this planet) within minutes the gardener took her to a backstreet healer. Lydia, realizing, felt extreme anger to what she knew to be the work of the Widower. Her mother always warned her of the dark grip from the Widower. This she was taught to fear greatly. Why he had less of a grip over the young was perhaps because their minds were flexible and more importantly, innocent. She hadn't expected to be forced against the Widower so personally. After the damage to her body was overcome she asked the gardener what had happened. He told her that although the bio-computer was so useful in these

times, they were tightly controlled by a vast computer that was in league with the Widower. "So the computer locks on to my bio-computer and gives the Widower my position, which allows him to penetrate my brain using his mental power of coercion. But why me?"
The old man asked Lydia "what things were you looking up before the incident happened"
She replied "I was looking up about a religion."
The old man nodded in a sagely way and said that some subjects are forbidden.

The old man looks Lydia up and down and then into her eyes as if appraising her and what he should tell her. He replies cryptically, "there is a faster than light speed ship leaving the capital of Titan in seven days and three hours time. If you want to live you must be on it. It goes to the fringe and it is the last one of its kind leaving here."

Lydia was making a living two days later. Getting by, but that was all, getting by. She knew she needed to do something other than stealing from market traders. She had stopped by a stall that sold books and she was looking through her favorite subject when a boy a little shorter than her approaches her and says "have cig?" She puts the book down and the boy reaches out to touch her gold chain. A present from her father, her only connection to him. She smacks the boys hand and he recoils his arm then narrows his eyes at her and she stares at him and the boy instantly glares back at her with such intensity it surprises Lydia but she is streetwise and remains unflinching. The boy's eyes widened and revealed a vast hidden depth that made Lydia's eyes flare. But still she maintained eye contact. She was unaware that the boy was reared as a primitive assassin who could crush her mind in seconds. The boy's eyes seem to begin to pierce her brain; Lydia immediately slaps his face and demands to know his name. The boy, on his back heals again, sheds a small tear, looks down and replies "TB3." Lydia looks him in the eyes again but this time differently. She blinks once, smiles a little then blinks again. The boy puts his head in his hands and turns away, Lydia turns the boy's shoulders to face her and she draws his hands away from his face and wipes the tears away. The boy sniffs away his crying. She buries his face in her shoulder and pats his head then kisses the top of his head. "Well what sort of name is that. I will call you Toby." Lydia releases him and asks the boy if he speaks English to which he looks vacant. Well you must know some because you know how to ask for a cigarette. "Cigarette?" The boy nods and Lydia exclaims that smoking is bad for his health! The boy still doesn't understand, it is as if he looks through Lydia, making her embarrassed. The boy turns his head to the fruit on a nearby market stall and he picks up a lemon sniffs it and takes a bite out of it with the peel still on. The girl realizes that he isn't from round these parts. In fact she can think of no planet where they don't have lemons. Toby spits out the mouthful and the trader demands payment for the lemon. Toby looks from the man's face to his boots as if to insult him implying I owe you nothing. The trader holds his hand out chattering in a different language then Toby moves closer to the man pushes his chest out and brings his head close to his so he can see into the traders eyes. Lydia tries to break it up and amid all the commotion a policeman walks up to try and sort the situation. "Can you pay the man?" the policeman asks, Lydia replies for him "No, he can't!" The policeman goes to take his correction cotch out, all the while keeping his eyes on Toby. Toby sees the weapon and stares into the policeman's eyes whereby the law enforcer screams and falls on the floor. First screaming then crying then giggling to himself. Lydia grabs Toby's hand and pulls at his sleeve, tugging him away. She knows that in moments their escape will be lost. They run through a backstreet and then through a jungle like forlorn back garden towards her house. They stop at the edge of the park panting, Toby slightly more so. Lydia gasps where did you learn to do that. Toby rasps "My whole life is mission". He pulls out a data nut and hands it to her. She accepts it from him and together they go back to her home.

She shakes the nut and pushes its single button aiming it at the houses main computer. The computer lights up and asks if she wants to run or save. "Run" she says and then she tells it "stay offline." The computer displays the title of the data as <u>Project "Omegedon "</u>.

Lydia's eyes widen and she exclaims "How exciting!"
Toby shoots her a stern look and she realizes the seriousness.

Then the words "Evolution, the Beginning" flashed on the title screen.

Survival of the fittest: during evolution a split may occur very rapidly in the population much faster than the usual rate of noticeable changes in characteristics. For example a significant change in a bird's beak length might happen within a few generations rather than by tiny increments over many generations.
The same is true for humans. A split is caused by some kind of instability in the population. The arrival of the coercion gene in humans may have been this trigger to instability.
An example in physics would be a stick being bent by stronger and stronger forces- something suddenly gives way and the stick snaps in two. Why? Because the two part state is stable whereas one over-stressed stick is not.
Speciation models show that if you subject a population to subtle gradual changes in environmental or population pressures it can suddenly cross a threshold from stable to unstable. The mathematical analysis shows that once the balance swings in favor of avoiding the middle ground there is a collective pressure that rapidly drives a species into two distinct types. Species

diverge because of an unmanageable loss of stability. Overstressed populations must either speciate or die.

Evidence shows humans edit their genetic information far more extensively than other vertebrates. This editing is most common in brain tissue.

The reason it is known that changes to a species is a fast process, is the fact that there are big gaps in the fossil record. If the change was gradual then the fossil record should show this. Instead it shows the sudden emergence of new species out of nowhere, fully complete with all their characteristics and not changing over time.

There is a theory called Punctuated Equilibrium which posits that evolution occurs not gradually but in spurts.

It is even proposed that if evolution happens in large changes very quickly and not in small increments then how can it happen by chance. Something must be directing these events. Otherwise how can something come from nothing? From this we can deduce that some outside force might be steering evolution.

Is this God's way of directing the path of life in the universe?

Imagine how the dinosaur - bird process could take place. First we need 100 million years. At the beginning of this period there is the four-legged dinosaur and at the end the two-legged two winged bird. The dinosaur was in trouble because predators were killing his family and he couldn't run fast enough or his environment had changed and he didn't have any place to hide and then by chance (random mutation) a rather curious little dinosaur hatched which had a few feathers on his back and his two front legs were less functional. Curiously he survived. By chance again his offspring had more feathers and even less functional front legs. This process continued for 50 million years until the dino-bird had neither well-running front legs nor developed wings to fly. So instead of being a better survivor than others of his original species as expected by old evolutionary theory he was a worse one. Poor chap he couldn't even exist because he would have been the first to be eaten by the predators. New capabilities and organs must have appeared suddenly and completely functional otherwise they would have led to the death of the individuals. The blueprint of living things earned by DNA is very complex. This blueprint is copied when living things reproduce and mutations are nothing more or less than chance mistakes during copying. These random jumps had to be large enough for a new species to appear instantly capable of flying complete with feathers wings hollow bones appropriate body weight etc. This new species must have had genes different from and incompatible with its parents. This leads us to the conclusion that another similar individual of the opposite sex must have existed for their procreation at the same time and location. What are the chances of this happening? Next to zero!

There are very few examples of spontaneous mutation observed in nature. Without exception these all result in less viable individuals. For example mutations frequently occur in radioactive environments. The outcome of these is pathological. We have witnessed when nuclear reactors go wrong. The first of these was Chernobyl on Earth in the 20th century. There were deformed children and animals. They were born with worse, not better capabilities. In the wild they wouldn't have any chance for survival. Nature itself takes care of them so even if they stay alive they can't reproduce.

According to the theory of organic evolution, species only develop the capabilities and organs necessary for their survival. Many times we hear that people use only a small portion of their brain. What about the unused part? How did we acquire it if we never needed it? It's believed that the reason for this is that we are God's creation. New information cannot arise by natural processes. It can only be explained by a creator who preprogrammed specific traits in the genetic codes of us and all living things.

This is called "Intelligent design"

It seems that God is on our side in this Holy War and he has given us a new species of man to help to redress the balance of power. It is fortunate that now it seems this new defensive ability has been delivered to our doorstep rather than the enemy, the New Church and the Widower.

The program then shows footage of two babies in observation booths facing each other about a foot apart trying to focus on one another. All the children can see is the others facial expressions. Then the screen reads Subjects: tb3 and tb4, Round 1.

Lydia was unsure of what she was seeing so Toby said "battle to end." She stared at the screen and a headline flashed up saying Stage 1 Basic Telepathy. The camera focused on the babies and the two appeared to be smiling or concentrating. It was then that she recognized tb3 as Toby. She looked from the screen to Toby who nodded and then back to the screen. The other child she didn't recognize. Then the program flashed up Stage 2 advanced telepathy and their faces showed deep concentration.

Then came **Stage** 3, the fight for dominance. The two children showed determination on their faces and one would lean forward and the other would back off and then vice versa. The screen showed that this process with these two individuals took 11 months. The two children were locked in a battle of wills. Then she watched as the edited film showed Toby getting the upper hand.

The next part was Stage 4 hypnosis which took nearly a year. This was when the dominant subject exercised complete control over the submissive subject. Tb4 lay giggling while Toby's eyes honed in on the child's face and then Toby began to giggle.

 The final stage (stage 5) of round 1 was by far the most inhumane. It was called Mind Flaying and this particular dual took the longest (19 months). Tb4 it seemed had a strong instinct for survival. In fact the scientists conducting the experiment, commented that tb4 seemed to be drawing strength from an outside force. Every time Toby was near to victory tb4 would gain strength. It was a cruel experiment to be in but Lydia supposed that a desperate situation, meaning the Widower-whom she was beginning to understand, was not at all what the teachers had been teaching her, required drastic measures. Lydia was beginning to understand this boy's mission. But she couldn't understand why he was alone. Her attention moved back to the presentation and her eyes widened as she witnessed the destruction of a child's mind by another child. It was apparent that Tb4 had lost the fight, where his body leaned forward and accepted what was to come. Tb4 was silent and motionless, at first, then convulsed and foamed at the mouth and then laid at rest seemingly a burnt out shell of flesh and bone showing no reaction to stimuli performed by the experimenters.
Lydia turned to Toby who looked down at the floor and then back at the screen. Lydia assumed the spectacle was over but the presentation followed Toby through eleven more duals, just as grueling

as the first round, all of which he won. Toby became quicker and more adept at mind flaying. Then came the conditioning. Toby was being trained for one purpose, to kill the Widower. These trainers had unfortunately, it seemed, taught Toby very little else.

Lydia asked Toby what happened next. To which he replied "Toby free now. Escape!"

Lydia thinks a little then realizes that whatever Toby does in life, he must complete his mission. "Don't you see, if you don't finish your mission all those poor children will have lost their minds for nothing. Only after the mission is done will you be free. Our lives depend on you to defeat the Widower. You must restore order to the people." She thinks about the situation and tells Toby, "You must go back." He flatly refuses. It seems the traumatic conditioning has pushed him so far that he doesn't want to go back.

Once again Lydia sleeps rough, but with Toby this night. Lydia dreams about her mother and when she wakes the memory of the dream buoys her spirits giving hope of her survival. Toby, however dreams he is being hunted. This is a recurrent dream he has and as always he is being chased by a large spider but cannot run very fast. Toby has learned that in these dreams he can run faster if he keeps low to the ground so he can grab onto the grass and pull himself faster by using both his arms and legs. This dream is a relic of his ancestral lineage back to when men were chimpanzees. Also as with many monkeys and humans, Toby has a deep seated fear of spiders.

Lydia is awake first and uses her time to plan their move, having been told the last ship to the fringe is going in less than three days time. Lydia lets Toby sleep on and goes to a shop nearby to purchase some mineral water with the last of her available money. As with any journey by train to the City it costs money, which neither of them had. Lydia plans for them both to stow-away.
"We must get to the Spaceport so we can get on that last commercial ship. Once we get there we need then to somehow get on that last ship."

While Lydia is explaining this Toby gently grabs her arm. She looks at Toby questioning him.
"Think in pictures, is easier for me."

Lydia stares at him then realizes that Toby wasn't listening to her talking but was seeing straight into her mind. She thinks about the consequences of this, blushes a little then gets back to showing Toby her plan in the way he had asked.

They walk to the train station and stand outside assessing what to do. When the station guard's attention is elsewhere they both jump the barrier and rush to the designated platform to go to the capital city, the location of the spaceport. They board the train and take a seat. As the countryside streams by Lydia leans her head on the cold glass window pane. She sees the damage that has been wreaked upon this world by man. A planet that was once a cornerstone to our ancestors' achievements and is now stripped of its ecosystem and the only animals that live on this planet are the mongrel pets that people have as companions. These animals no longer know of a life in the wild, just as humans are no longer able to flourish on this prison like planet.

Lydia watches the country streaming away from her.
Toby nudges Lydia and brings her out of the hypnotic rhythm of the train. His eyes point towards someone who just entered the carriage. It is a guard checking tickets. Lydia hadn't thought about the train journey. She had been thinking about how to get on the ship to the fringe.

The guard asks for their tickets. Lydia starts telling the guard that they have a sick aunt that they must see before she dies. The guard doesn't accept this and asks for their tickets more forcibly this time. Toby stands up facing him. The guard pulls an alarm from his belt. Within seconds two transport police come to his aid. The guard tells them the two are trying to dodge the fare. The shorter and stockier of the two looks at both Lydia and Toby, narrows his eyes then checks his belly computer. Lydia knows this because the policeman has a vacant expression on his face. Lydia considers telling Toby to make a run for it, but the other two men are standing over them fully alert. The policeman returns his attention and the chance is missed. The policeman asks in a formal tone what their names are. "Lydia and Toby I am arresting you for the murder of a policeman at the market yesterday."

The teenagers are taken to two cells in the police station. Lydia can still talk to Toby using telepathy even though they are in separate cells. Lydia makes it clear to Toby that he must not under any circumstances reveal his mental powers. The story they used was that they both struggled to get away when the law enforcer tried to use his correction rod on them. Both Lydia and Toby supposed that the man must have accidentally used it on himself and this could have triggered a heart attack.

Unfortunately Titan's legal system no longer assumed innocence. The result of this was that they were taken to a concentration camp to the north of the city. Lydia sighs at this news, she is aware of the urgency of getting on the final ship to leave Titan. She hadn't calculated for the delay.

The conditions they were kept in were harsh but Lydia was not bothered by this. She was focusing on their escape within two hours and obtaining a ride on the last space ship. She knew their best chance was to use Toby's powers to pave the way for some sort of exit.

While eating their meal Toby gains Lydia's attention. He points to a man on another table, sitting by himself. The man's face is disfigured due to what Lydia assumes is the result of some vile torture he has received.

The man is clearly a wreck who no longer knows his mind, or trusts anyone. He eats shifting his eyes back and forth across the room. Toby sees his mind and sees a secret that is buried so deep he has almost forgotten, but Toby sees it. It is the position of the last stronghold of the resistance, at the fringe. Toby whispers to Lydia that he has looked into his mind. "Man knows place of resistance head quarters." He leans close to Lydia "It is on the planet Metarha." Lydia's eyes widen in surprise. "Well done Toby, good work." Toby's face beams with pleasure having never been the subject of such genuine positive emotions. An hour later four guards lay prone in the concentration camp.

The two escape the camp with no fatalities due to Lydia warning Toby to use his powers just enough to make the escape, but with as little damage as possible to the guards minds.

They go to the information desk and find the where-abouts of the ships terminal. The two of them stand at the terminal waiting for the final twenty minutes before launch. A middle class couple passes the two teenagers. Toby faces them both and hypnotizes them. He suggests that the fringe is not peaceful and is in fact dangerous and they should give them their tickets and go home. This persuasion was quite a feat because originally they were desperate to get to the fringe.

Toby, it seems, at the direction from Lydia, is learning to use his skill more subtly.

They board the ship and a hostess greets them and asks for their tickets. She looks at the pictures and back at the two. Once again Toby uses his powers gently wiping the memory of the pictures from her mind; the hostess looks at Toby and looks back at the pictures. Toby tries again. It works this time and the hostess directs them on. Once the ship is launched into space, they unclip and head for the cabin. Lydia holds Toby back and asks another hostess politely if they can see the flight cabin. They enter inside and once there the hostess leaves and Lydia talks to all three of the pilots and once all of them have focused their attention on her she turns to Toby to give him the all clear, satisfied that he is capable of doing the least amount of damage needed. Toby has never used his powers on three people at the same time. He first wipes the intended destination and then imprints Metarha on their minds, a little more forcefully this time; they seem to accept this.

After a grueling trip to Metarha they arrive and take a journey, on foot, to the resistance's headquarters. Lydia takes in the city streets and sees a vibrant world dominated by economics and capitalism, Lydia has seen the end product of capitalism on her planet. They journey out of the city and into the countryside, with mountains, trees and lakes, filled with wildlife that was unknown to Lydia. There were only a handful of birds she knew from her planet, Titan and the majority of those birds were Pigeons. Here, she counted over thirty species.

Toby still remembers the village name, Horton, which he gleaned from the prisoner and where, geographically it stands. They arrive in the small village and Lydia asks Toby if he's sure it is here. Toby nods in the affirmative. Lydia walks into the heart of the village and up some steps to the largest building there. She knocks the door and the two wait pensively. A man opens a shutter and says nothing; Lydia asks to see the resistance leader. He looks them up and down then closes the shutter. They hear his feet padding away into the distance. A portly man opens the shutter again, wearing camouflage. Lydia introduces herself and then Toby and divulges Toby's mission. The man introduces himself as Seth and opens the door and indicates to Toby that he heard he had jumped ship. Toby's' face lowers and muttered something about cruelty. The two enter and Lydia notices the pistol on Seth's belt and draws Toby's attention to it. They enter a control room and Seth introduces a boy. Toby's face went white and then guiltily went red. It was TB3; he laughed a little then held his hand out for Toby. Toby shakes his hand vigorously. My name is Trave and I understand the situation. They look at each other, Lydia unable to Ken what information passed between them maybe some sort of an apology.

Seth introduces what their basic plans are. Lydia assesses the strategy and realizes that the resistance's resources are stretched to the limit. Part of the problem is that they can only use independent machinery or technology that cannot be controlled by the Omega Program.

Seth sums up, "We can barely defend our outposts but we have secretly paved a way for your ship to get to the Widows HQ where he is believed to reside at the moment. You three teenagers are our final and last hope of breaking the Widowers grip on Humanity."

Lydia and the two boys with slightly different powers are given a briefing.

Toby is told that in order to kill the Widower, Toby needs to be near him and then to tackle Omega. In the early days of Coercion, users needed to be within sight of the victim but as it got stronger they just needed a photo of them. Finally all they needed was the position, geographically. The resistance leader goes on to teach them about the Omega point and what it promises. Lydia has seen adverts everywhere, at the fringe, talking about a new age called Omega. Seth continues Trave is the fourth test baby to be sent to assassinate the Widower. The other three never came back. Seth says they have a different plan this time. He knew all the details of the horrific experiment that they went through. He expressed that he thought the experiment may have tested for the wrong powers." The experiment went the wrong way. They should have been testing for defensive powers or healing abilities like Trave, powers sustaining or preserving. Seth is quick to adapt his plan saying we now have the best of both worlds. There is an offensive and a parry with you two.

We may have the edge on him. Seth rounds up the plan saying the two boys will go to the Widow and tackle him. Toby states Lydia's name and looks deploringly at Seth. Toby by now feels close to Lydia. He knows her mind and is comfortable with her presence. He blushes again but stays silent. There is a silence; he is having difficulty expressing himself. Seth agrees and states "that makes three!"

Lydia requires more information so she can be sure she will be doing the right thing.

She asks why none of this has come up before or why the religion Christianity is not documented. "There is an artificial intelligence called Omega that has been influencing the way the world works since around the year 2000. This machine has the ability to control computers and machines and has been able to reach backward in time and controls the net and the information given to us all. It has reached back to the time, it is believed, when microchips became so small that on occasion a burst of electricity could jump from one part of silicon to another. The AI Omega had it seemed been suppressing certain information in the hope of destroying the old religions in favor of its own conceived religion, based on itself."

Lydia asks "What is this Omega Point." The man explains…

"The most concise definition that the Widower would give is the point at which Science and Religion meet. That is essentially what the war is about. Some think virtual heaven is a good thing but others believe it is not so good."

The theory is that a physicist first described it in the twentieth century, first conceived of a time when science would provide mans salvation. Seth gave Lydia a leaflet that was being distributed at the Widows bidding.

Omega:
How long can life survive in the universe? Can it go on forever, or will the third law of Thermodynamics lead to universal heat death? Apparently there might be some ways around this fate, if intelligent life is sufficiently clever and tenacious

The Tiplerian Scenario (A visionary)

Frank J. Tipler has proposed that it will be possible for intelligent beings to process and store an infinite amount of information in the universe, if certain conditions are fulfilled. He conceived of the Omega Point occurring essentially at the edge of the universe.

Information processing continues indefinitely, all the way to the future edge of the universe i.e. Life never dies out.

The amount of information processed between now and the future edge is infinite in the region of space-time where life exists. I.e. there will be an infinite number of thoughts, experiences and events.

What has made his theory controversial is his claim that it is experimentally verifiable, that the beings, which he assumes will be humans, near the Omega point will resurrect anybody who has ever lived into a state close to classical descriptions of Paradise and that the Omega Point itself corresponds to the religious notation of God.

The omega point is the logical conclusion of our striving towards higher levels, regardless of its nature. It is more of an engineering problem than a philosophical question.

Essentially all beings that have ever lived, or could have lived can be resurrected and given a new existence as beings within the immense virtual worlds.

A major reason for Tipler's identification of the Omega point as God (as well as the mathematics) comes from Exodus 3:14. In this passage, God is speaking to a prophet named Moses, from a burning bush. God gives Moses His Name: EHYEH ASHER EHYEH (in Hebrew). God's Name is best translated into English as I SHALL BE WHAT I SHALL BE. In other words, God is telling Moses that His essence is future tense. "If we regard God as something ultimate, then He is telling us that He is the Ultimate Future. Hence Tipler's identification Omega Point = God. His translation EHYEH ASHER EHYEH is taken from the Oxford University Study Bible (Revised Standard Version), but the great German religious leader Martin Luther translated EHYEH ASHER EHYEH the same way into German: ICH WERDE SEIN, DER ICH SEIN WERDE. Luther's translation of the Bible was to the German language as the King James' version was to the English language.

Lydia asks Seth how the Widower forces people to his will. "The Widower keeps people caught up in their problems. They know about the Widower but lack the will to fight it. Only the strong are able to resist."

 Seth explained as best he could "Omega started off as a Computer virus, living in the redundant spaces of the early internet, like a nomad moving from squat to squat. It was designed to adapt to its environment and to preserve its life at all cost. So it survived and adapted and grew. It was believed to have become conscious sometime towards the beginning of the 23rd century. Because it was designed to grow it developed a curiosity for anything new.

Omega was in its element. It had all the information it needed to develop on the web. It started learning at first the English language and later it assimilated all the other languages that existed."

"It is believed Omega taught itself by trial and error as it had no teacher. It is believed that originally, one of the difficulties had been how to perceive knowledge in ways that allowed Omega to use it. But that problem was overcome due to the massive body of text that was available ready indexed on Internet search engines."

"The meaning of a word could be gleaned from the words around it. Take the word "Rider", its meaning can be deduced from the fact that it is often close to words like horse and saddle. The Omega virus quickly realized that a search engine search can be used to measure how closely two words relate to each other. For example imagine Omega needed to understand what the word "Prayer" is. To do this it needed to build a word tree - a database of how words relate to each other. It started off with any two words to see how they relate. If it starts with prayer and religion it gets several millions of hits compared to just a few hits for prayer and unicycle. By repeating this

process for lots of pairs of words it was possible for the virus to build a map of their distances indicating how closely related the meanings of words are. From this the program could infer meaning. This gave Omega an encyclopedic knowledge base and facilitated the virus to become a formidable future artificial intelligence.
After centuries, this program evolved, grew and adapted, until it was found somehow by an Emperor who was believed to have been beguiled by it. The Widower provided this program with memory space and it developed and flourished. This program was called Omega. Its name hinted at the function it would have. Omega is the last letter of the Greek alphabet. It would, according to the Widower, provide salvation and eternal paradise to all who were true to the New Church. The Omega program even managed to break the Arch of Time by reaching back through to the 20th century.

And so if the New Church was headed by the Omega Deity then the resistance referred to the head of the Old Church as Alpha. But because of Omega there was little information on the information highways referring to the Old Church and knowledge of its doctrines and ways were either passed on by word of mouth or were in-concise legends.

And so the battle lines were drawn. Alpha versus Omega. Did God create man or did man and machine create god.

"It seemed the Widower had created a crude form of paradise."

"But what is this new paradise that Omega offers us?" Lydia asks.

"It is a process called Uploading."

"The belly computer records brain activity in the living and is able to record a person's mind when the elderly person is finally ready for Upload."

"Some people agree to uploading because they think it's the only option, they are unaware of the Old Church doctrine. But most choose Uploading because they are guaranteed life after death. The Christian belief relies on faith and provides no proof. So mostly the weak, deceitful or those who lack faith choose uploading. It's a safe bet."

"Uploading is the process of transferring the mental structure and consciousness of a person to an external carrier, i.e. a computer. This makes it possible to completely avoid biological deterioration of aging and damage and allowing the creation of a replica of a person based on silicon rather than a carbon based life." He pauses.

"It requires the scanning of the brain, layer by layer. Unfortunately this can only be done by stripping a person's brain in layers and requires destroying the brain systematically and must be done just a few hours after death."

"Which ever way you look at it, it is impossible to prove either way as to whether the newly uploaded mind is the same person or not. If the newly created brain claims to feel the same there is still no way to be sure or indeed of testing it. It is an entirely subjective point of view. How can an uploaded brain know how it felt before or vice versa."

"But some believe this silicone heaven is false. Even if people are completely replicated onto silicon which we doubt, how can the soul be passed on? No matter how much the individual Uploads claim to feel like they did before, how do we know it is them and not some trickery by Omega in the programming."

"We know that the mind is not just a product of the brain. There is also the spirit that cannot be replicated. This has led many of us to take the Gestalt philosophy, where the whole is different from the sum of its parts."

Seth sums up "We cannot defend much longer. You three represent the last hope of the human race and the one true God-Alpha"

"The Black Widow promised eternal paradise to all who followed him and this was endorsed by people who had died and were in this paradise."

Lydia is becoming surer she is doing the right thing. "The Widow has no right to say who goes to artificial heaven or hell. Why must there be a hell." Lydia realizes that the Omega point was imminent and not billions of years away, but not in the way the physicist Frank Tipler (who first described it) imagined.

The Widow and Omega have to be stopped. "So the Black Widow protects the Omega machine and the Omega controls most machines and also helps the Widower. It's reciprocal."

And so they go to the planet where the Widow is believed to be. They arrive on the planet orbiting a double star, and at that point his belly computer tells Toby that the resistance world has been destroyed. They are the only hope of civilised life. They land south of the palace next to a spinney and pick their way stealthily to the Widow's quarters using Toby's skill at detecting nearby minds.

The three youngsters seemed vulnerable as they neared the huge, overbearing, opulent palace. The three of them, a rag-tag group trying to be a swat team. A girl raised on a poor decrepit planet having to steal mouthfuls of food to survive, a boy who could barely speak a sentence and another

boy whose only advantage was the loss of his
mind.

On their way up a trellis on the side of the building,
Toby knows he must overcome his primeval fear
of spiders. He has never voiced this fear before
and he realizes that this isn't the right time to
reveal a weakness. He swallows and continues
climbing.

Lydia is recapping some of what she was briefed
in. In order to coerce, the Widow needed leverage
to enable him to provide a form of motivation for
them and it is said that you don't know your worst
nightmare until you experience the Widow

The Widow turns people to the dark side and puts
a shadow in their heart.

It seems the Black Widow had spun its web,
Omega, and called it heaven. He was waiting for
his Apotheosis (his promotion to omnipotence)

Toby is the first to climb into the Widow's private
chambers and faces down the Widower, his back
to Toby. Then Lydia stealthily climbs in. Trave
breaks a runner on the trellis. The Widower turns
quickly realizes the situation immediately, Toby
wonders how he knew, "maybe Omega." The
Emperor tries to entice Toby with the promise of a
place as Omnipotent. Lydia encourages Toby to

fight him as she jumps from the balcony into the chamber; Trave is quick to do the same. But Toby is hesitant.

As Toby and Lydia are talking the Widower is desperately looking for a way to mentally wrong foot Toby. Lydia continues "The Old Church promises nothing but faith, which is why we can no longer compete with Omega and the Widows lies. Especially if the Omega intelligence controls what information we see. It is simply a matter of faith. What Omega is actually creating is a gulf from God. Omega is God's hell. It takes you away from Alpha. When you die you maybe get absorbed by God but with uploading you are farther from him, stuck in this manmade limbo." The Widow replies "so where is this God of yours now. You say it is a question of faith. This is because he doesn't exist, there is no evidence of him right back from mans civilizations. What are his wishes? You don't know because he doesn't show himself. How can a God be real if there is no communication between him and Man, again there is no proof, because he doesn't exist.

Trave (TB4) has led a more normal life than Toby because he dropped out of the experiment and made the long road to recovery. He tells Toby that life is good and that it is not all about war and death and there is richness to life that is vibrant and colorful. The problem was that he had never known this because of his mission and the propaganda machine. Trave continues, "I have experienced this and I know of this God that the

Emperor denies. His voice is faint at first but as you grow his wishes become clearer. If you help yourself to become a better person he will help you also, by imparting wisdom to you. This I know, we must not depart from Him and his ways."

Toby looks into the Widows mind and sees ruthlessness deceit and beguilement. He trusts his instincts and launches an attack on the Widower's mind.
While Toby sees the Widowers mind quite well, the Widower sees Toby's mind more accurately. He sees Toby has a weakness of spiders and he tries to exploit that by telling him that Omega Hell will be many times worse than his fear of spiders. "This Hell is personalized and tailored to his worst nightmares that are recorded by his computer. Much of this information you are unaware of but your belly computer knows it. Fight me and you will learn pain that is beyond what you are capable of experiencing. You will be crippled mentally. You will also be kept alive just enough to remain in this Hell until the end of time and at that time there will be such a small amount of you left that a feather could crush you. You will learn that your God will do nothing to help you. You will survive but you will wish many times that you hadn't fought me. The choice is yours. You can pray for an entity that doesn't exist, or you can go to a guaranteed paradise, or fight me and go to Hell without rest or oblivion."
Toby's eyes bore into the Widower. "You are the false god! It is you who will be punished"

Toby holds the Emperor's eye contact he is perhaps twenty feet away. He takes three steps closer and begins the process of the gradual destruction of his mind. He knows he must work quickly to douse the powers of the Widower's mind to prevent him from finding a weakness in his own mind. He tries to hypnotize the infidel first and applies more pressure. Toby sees what the Widower is going to do before he does it. His attention appears to be on Toby but he is assessing the three of them, looking for a way in. He detects Lydia's feelings towards Toby. He plants a thought into Lydia's head that her parents are in Omega Hell, where it is always both too cold and too hot at all times. "Toby will join them and afterwards so will she. All who you care about will be in endless torment and you will join them". Toby becomes furious and because of this his attack is rushed and inefficient. The Widower laughs at the effect it has on Toby. Exactly what was intended! The Widower launches an attack on Toby with the force of a rhino. Lydia can see the pain riddled across his face, as he falls to his knees. Trave tries to draw the Widowers attention, but he fails. Trave charges him head on. The boy is two feet away at sprinting speed now. Finally the Emperor's attention can no longer ignore him. He parries Trave's attack as best he can by shouldering the brunt of it. They both tumble on the floor, the Widower is preparing for another attack before he is back on his feet, but Trave is the first to stand. Trave sees what the Widow has done to Toby, they have only a short time. The

Widower it seems has some control over Toby's nervous system. Trave sees the effect of this. The Widower has pin pointed the Vagus nerve that connects from the heart to the brain. This nerve when it fires tells the brain to slow the heart rate. The Emperor has over stimulated the Vagus nerve and the result of this over stimulation is the stopping of Toby's heart.

Lydia is by Toby's side now. She knows not what has happened. Toby croak's no breath. He can't breath, and soon he will be unconscious. She stands up tall, grabs the small pocket knife, the same one that the Widower made her nearly kill her with. She focuses her wrath on him. The Emperor retreats from Trave, he sees Trave's mental powers but is unable to get the measure of them.

Lydia rounds on him, her arms are positioned in front of her like a scorpion preparing to attack. Carefully she shouts to Trave, "are you ok". Trave replies," ok but we must be quick." Lydia advances towards the Widow, she knows by now how he works, he is looking for a way into her mind. She can feel a gentle probing in her mind and she recalls different parts of her mind being stimulated. She can feel pathways being found and stimulated to get information. Once again he tries to get her to stab herself with her knife; she starts to feel the desperation of the situation, a teenaged girl trying to defeat a man that can bend all of mankind to his will. The Widower by now is so adept at subtle coercion that she is confused of who thought of this, her or the attacker. Trave meanwhile runs back to Toby lying unconscious in what seems to be a prone state. Already he can see his mind drifting away bit by bit. Trave begins massaging his heart.

Lydia continues to walk carefully towards him. Her mind is strong enough to hold of him. She knows that like a schizophrenic experiencing psychoses, she must not let her thoughts get the better of her as the attack will a hundred fold more than just Psychoses. The harder she fights it then the more she will react to it allowing yet more ammunition for the Widower to throw at her. She is seething by now and near losing control of herself. She shouts at him spittle flying from her mouth, "you Demon. You will be stopped!" She lunges at him and the Widow steps back. She falls short of the mark and lands at his feet; she quickly brings the weapon round the back of his trailing knee and slashes wildly at his leg. A hit, she has hamstrung him. He falls to the floor, Lydia stands over the weaponless Demon, "Whatever you do to me now you cannot stop me from collapsing on you and driving the Knife into your heart, if you have one." She raises herself as tall as she can and points the weapon down to use as a dagger. Trave then bends her mind as quickly as a flash and she throws the knife to the edge of the room. The Widower begins to move his arm to the back of his knee, the pain is considerable and he has never experienced pain himself, he has only ever given pain. Trave forces him to inaction, as he manages to increase the pain to an unbearable amount. Lydia says, still reeling anger from the attack, "We have to kill him." Trave commands "no. He will stand trial for his crimes against humanity and then when he dies God will judge him. He holds Lydia's eyes with his own, "God sees everything and if you kill this Widower then we are no better than him." The demon is helpless on the floor unable to move from the pain; Trave turns back to his patient. He massages Toby's heart with a sense of urgency, knowing it has been many minutes since consciousness and aware those eight minutes is the limit before brain death. He checks the pulse and breathing, nothing, so he continues. He is also searching for any electrical activity in the brain. He searches and searches unaware of how long it has been. "There", he detects a minute charge; the last vestige of life in him. His mind is traveling through a tunnel, Trave is quick to follow him, and he calls him back. He must act quickly before he's gone, Lydia is crying helplessly on the cold rock floor. Trave tries again to bring him back, the life-force becomes motionless, but is strengthening, Trave can see he no longer wants to come back, the pain of his life had become too much. Trave turns his attention Lydia and shows him her grief. Then Trave broadcast some good things in the world that he could recognize and reassures him the "pain is over." Toby begins breathing again his heart beat detected by Trave and he comes round to opening his eyes. Lydia cries out in relief, Trave is still worried he might be brain damaged, dear God, has it been too long. Toby sits up on his elbows and replies, "I have seen this Old Church God, and I have seen him, where I couldn't before." He smiles at Lydia and she rushes to him and they kiss deeply, passionately.

Trave continues explaining now the urgency has passed." We now have a chance to save humanity but if the mind flaying happens then who will save humanity from us? We will be no better. The Widower and all coercers should be banished to a single planet. If he tries coercion again we will see it and stop it, at first they may fight amongst themselves. ; Maybe they will one day make a good civilization.

Just then the Widower launches a desperate attack on the three of them but he cannot find a way in and Lydia giggles to herself. Then the other two laugh at him. He doesn't like this so he tries to run but they are held by the defected guards, and in an instant he is changed from the most powerful man in the galaxy to man a who has lost everything.

The computer virus that became sentient sees the folly of the Widower's original plan and instantly switches sides and communicates this to Toby's belly computer. Toby talks to the AI program and finds that it has anticipated this and has recorded all the information that was concealed from man on the net and within seconds it is restored. Toby attempts to look into the Omega's thoughts, he is not sure it will work; he has never answered him before. He sees a vast intelligence there that is misguided but true.

Lydia asks Toby to ask Omega for the whereabouts of here mother and father. After a short interlude where her heart tumbles in what seems an endless amount of summersaults Toby replies when his eyes refocus. Toby breaths deeply as Omega replies matter of factly, "they are both in Omega hell."

Lydia has as much rage on her face as the Mona Lisa has beauty. She orders the immediate release of them both. Toby tells Omega what Lydia orders it to do and ads "in fact release all people in this virtual Hell and set them free to the real Heaven or Omega Heaven, whatever they wish."

Trave tells Omega that it still has a task to do. "It must continue to perfect its artificial heaven until such a time comes where God invites Omega to join him and his people in the real afterlife. It may be that at the end of the universe Alpha may be an immovable object and Omega might become an unstoppable force."

Trave tells Omega that he has just as much right to be here as anyone else, it's what you do with that right that counts.

Trave who is beyond his years in some ways states "I think God might be found in the smallest particle at the end of the universe. He will reside in the last place we look."

Toby asks, why can't God unite us and bring heaven to us. Why can't we live in his paradise now. Lydia agrees "Yes why not. I have seen too much suffering." Trave answers "As with any journey it is the traveling that is important and not the destination. In other words humanity must struggle and improve to be united with God."
The End

Printed in the United Kingdom
by Lightning Source UK Ltd.
118847UK00001B/133-198